Liz Pearson is a Registered Dietitian and an award-winning p
al speaker with a passion for peanut butter sandwiches and a
love for chocolate. She runs The Pearson Institute of Nut
Fitness where she translates the science of nutrition into fun and con-
sumer-friendly language.

Liz Pearson lives in Toronto, Canada with her husband and daughter.

When in doubt, eat broccoli!

by

Liz Pearson, R.D.

A Denise Schon Book

Penguin Books

Dedication

This book is dedicated to my husband Rick, who forever encourages me to follow my dreams and to my beautiful daughter Chelsea, who brings a whole new level of happiness and wonderment to my life.

A Denise Schon Book

Penguin Books
Published by the Penguin Group
Penguin Books Canada Ltd, 10 Alcorn Avenue, Toronto, Ontario, Canada M4V 3B2
Penguin Books Ltd, 27 Wrights Lane, London W8 5TZ, England
Penguin Books USA Inc., 375 Hudson Street, New York, New York 10014, U.S.A.
Penguin Books Australia Ltd, Ringwood, Victoria, Australia
Penguin Books (NZ) Ltd, cnr Rosedale and Airborne Roads, Albany, Auckland 1310,
    New Zealand

Penguin Books Ltd, Registered Offices: Harmondsworth, Middlesex, England

Published in Penguin Books, 1998
Copyright © Liz Pearson, 1998
All rights reserved

Cataloguing-in-Publication Data

Pearson, Liz
        When in doubt, eat broccoli!

ISBN 0-14-026751-4

1. Nutrition. 2. Food. I. Title.
TX355.P42 1998   613.2   C97-931757-6

Design by Counterpunch/Linda Gustafson
Production editor Anna Barron
Cover photograph by Steve Rochon of the Foto Salon
Manufactured in Canada by Tri-Graphic Printing

Visit Penguin Canada's web site at **www.penguin.ca**

10 9 8 7 6 5 4 3 2 1

Contents

Top Ten Reasons That This Book Is for You   3

Top Three Things to Remember on the Road to Healthy Eating   6

Chapter One   Fat...the Good, the Bad and the Ugly   7

Chapter Two   Eat Fruits and Vegetables by the Truckload   17

Chapter Three   Be A Whole-Grain, High-Fibre Feaster   29

Chapter Four   Where's the Beef? (or Chicken, or Pork?)   43

Chapter Five   Be a Fish Eater   51

Chapter Six   Have Eggs Instead?   57

Chapter Seven   More Beans, Please!   61

Chapter Eight   Sometimes I Feel Like a Nut   69

Chapter Nine   Take a Ride on the Low-fat Milky Way   73

Chapter Ten   To Be or Not to Be...a Vegetarian   81

Chapter Eleven   It's Snack Time   85

Chapter Twelve   Desserts Make Life More Fun!   95

Chapter Thirteen   The Beverage Story   101

Chapter Fourteen   Pass the Sugar, Hold the Salt   115

Chapter Fifteen   Slim, Trim and Healthy   125

Chapter Sixteen   The Pill-Popping Question   137

Chapter Seventeen   Life in the Fast Lane   143

Chapter Eighteen   Children and Healthy Eating   157

Top Twelve Rules of Healthy Eating   165

The Best of the Best Recipes   167

Author's Acknowledgments

First and foremost I would like to thank Denise Schon for believing in this book and for ensuring every aspect of this project was well managed and of the highest quality. Thanks also to Anna Barron who cheerfully helped with everything from manuscript revisions to recipe testing.

Thanks to Jackie Kaiser and the rest of the team from Penguin for their commitment and dedication to this project. May this book mark the beginning of a successful launch into the nutrition/cookbook arena. Thanks to Jennifer Glossop for her outstanding work in editing the manuscript. She managed to clarify and encapsulate my ideas without ever losing my overall meaning or objectives. Thanks to Linda Gustafson for her extensive design work. The design required creativity, patience and skill, all of which she demonstrated beautifully.

Thanks to Alison Fryer, from the Cookbook Store, as well as Shelley Chambers, Stephanie Fox and Nancy MacIver, all of whom played an important role in the recipe selection process. Most importantly, thanks to the many talented people and organizations who contributed the recipes that appear in this book including Anne Lindsay, Bonnie Stern, Elizabeth Baird and the team from Canadian Living, Margaret Howard, Marjorie Hollands, Ellie Top, Kay Spicer, Monda Rosenberg, Frances Berkoff, Janet and Greta Podleski, Lynn Roblin, Bev Callaghan, Vesanto Melina, Lucy Waverman, Rose Reisman, Jan Main, Rose Murray, Nancy Enright, Heather Howe, Nestlé Canada, the Ontario Turkey Producers Marketing Board, the Beef Information Centre and the Tufts University Health & Nutrition Letter.

Thanks to the many dietitians who reviewed the manuscript from beginning to end. A special thanks to Suzanne Hendricks, Fran Berkoff and Cathy Camelon for their insightful comments, wonderful ideas and helpful suggestions.

Thanks to my dad who exemplifies excellence in his own career and inspires me to do my best, and to my mom who has been there for me always. Last but not least, a very special thank you to my wonderful friend and sister, Jenny. Not only did she read each and every chapter while still "hot off the press", she also provided a tremendous amount of support and encouragement along the way. To her I am truly grateful.

Top Ten Reasons That This Book Is for You

1. *It's Not about Eating Tofu for Breakfast* This book is not about eating tofu and bean sprouts for breakfast. It's about making simple changes in your lifestyle, based on your likes and dislikes. It's not about being a gourmet cook. It's about putting some basic principles to work when you eat at home or on the run. It's not about eliminating chocolate from your diet. It's about balance and moderation. In other words, this book is for real people who want suggestions for real life in the real world.

2. *It Can Significantly Influence Your Health* It's incredible. Every day new studies indicate that what you eat can greatly affect your health. Your risk of heart disease, cancer, high blood pressure and diabetes – four of the leading causes of death – can be significantly reduced by changing what you put in your mouth. The U.S. National Cancer Institute has even said that eight out of ten cancers have a nutrition/diet link. In other words, healthy eating is well worth the effort. To make it easy, this book identifies those foods that are the most nutritious. More specifically, the "Super Nutrition Tips" show you how to add more nutrition to everyday meals. The "Bronze, Silver and Gold Snacking List" identifies your best snacking options. And the "Top Ten List of Fruits and Vegetables" shows you how to get the biggest bang for your nutritional buck.

3. *It Makes the Complicated Seem Simple* The world of healthy eating is

filled with a mish-mash of mumbo-jumbo. Confusing terms like mono-unsaturated fats and polyunsaturated fats are thrown around with abandon. To add to the confusion the rules seem to change with the weather – one day it's margarine, the next day it's butter. Last but not least, we are bombarded with a never-ending stream of food myths and misconceptions. Well, it's time to take the mumbo out of jumbo, the mish out of mash. It's time to talk about healthy eating in simple terms with simple language. The truth is, healthy eating doesn't have to be so hard.

4. *It Has Great-Tasting Recipes*   Many people still equate "low fat" with "no taste." This book is here to change that point of view and challenge that assumption. How? First, through "Taste Tips," helpful suggestions to make good food taste better. Second, with a collection of the "Best of the Best" recipes from some of the top cookbook authors of today. With everything from Sweet Potato Salad to Bail-Out Bean Burritos, Apple Breakfast Bars to Broccoli Pesto Fettuccine, Herb Roasted Chicken to Modern Mashed Potatoes – all you have to do is open your mind (and your mouth).

5. *It Understands Your Busy Lifestyle*   If you lead a busy life, this book is for you. You can read it all at once or pick and choose among the chapters. And that's not all. This book is loaded with "Time Tips" and page after page of easy and efficient ways to save time at the supermarket and in the kitchen. For example, the list of "Top Ten Convenience Foods" makes shopping for quick, nutritious meals a breeze. The "Top Ten Fast-Food Survival Tips" is great when grabbing a quick meal away from home. Indeed, this book is filled with so much "timely" advice that by taking the time to read it, you'll actually have more time on your hands.

6. *It Shows You Where the Fat Is*   We all want to cut back on fat, both to reduce the damage caused by artery-lining saturated fats and to avoid the calories that all types of fat provide. This book makes fat-cutting easy. Graphs and charts clearly show the fat content of various foods, from lasagna to croissants, from Big Macs to large fries. In addition, numerous "Reduce the Fat" tips provide simple suggestions for reducing the fat in many of the foods you know and love.

7. *It Makes Weight Control Achievable*   Excess body weight is a growing problem for adults and children alike – hardly surprising in our world

where eating is easy and active living is not required. This book provides a realistic and enjoyable approach to weight loss. Long-term success is the ultimate goal. Ice cream is allowed (although frozen yogurt is highly recommended), and deprivation is forbidden. It's about eating when you're hungry and stopping when you're full. It's about identifying your weaknesses and building on your strengths. Best of all, it's a diet based on health.

8. *It Makes Active Living Easy*   Wouldn't it be nice to experience the extraordinary benefits of active living without feeling you have to be an Olympic athlete? Wouldn't it be nice to know that because today you cut the grass, or took a walk to the corner store, you made a significant difference in your overall health? Well, it's easier to reap the rewards of physical activity than previously thought. This book will show you how. It contains helpful tips on getting started and lots of suggestions for staying motivated. It's fun. It's easy. And better still, it will get you hooked for life.

9. *It Answers the Questions You Most Frequently Ask*   Vitamin supplements – should I take one? Alcohol – a drink a day? Sugar substitutes – are they safe? Salt and high blood pressure – what's the link? Eggs and cholesterol – what's the latest? Butter or margarine – which is better? Here are the answers to all those questions, and more. From antioxidants to olive oil, this book provides the most up-to-the-minute research on the most popular topics. You'll understand what; you'll understand why; you'll understand how; and so much more.

10. *It Understands Your Love of Food*   George Bernard Shaw said it best: "There is no love sincerer than the love of food." Eating is, without question, one the greatest pleasures in life. I want you to celebrate your love of food. I want you to enjoy each and every delicious morsel you put in your mouth. You shouldn't feel guilty because you had cheesecake on Tuesday and ice cream on Sunday. Spinach and beet greens are not the only route to health. Life is meant for foods you love. Life is meant for living.

In a Nutshell...

Quite possibly, this is the most fun, practical and insightful healthy-eating book that you will ever read.

Top Three Things to Remember on the Road to Healthy Eating

1. *It's Okay to Eat Chocolate*   Healthy eating is not about whether you had a piece of chocolate today. In fact, healthy eating is not even about what you had for lunch today. Healthy eating is about the quality of your food choices overall. It's about enjoying a wide variety of foods in moderation. It's about balancing your higher-fat choices with lower-fat choices. It's about increasing your activity today, because you were less active yesterday. It's about eating more vegetables tomorrow, because you didn't eat many today. Healthy eating is about you and your lifestyle. It's about being realistic and sensible, and doing the best you can.

2. *Small Changes Equal Big Rewards*   You may not think that putting a little less butter on your bread makes much of a difference, but it does. You may not think that adding a couple of carrot sticks to your lunch is that significant, but it is. And you may not think that taking the stairs instead of the elevator can really improve your health, but it will. Big differences in your health do not require big changes in your lifestyle. Try one new healthy recipe each month. Eat one more fruit or vegetable each day. Use milk in your coffee instead of cream. No matter how small, no matter how simple, it all adds up to a healthier day.

3. *Take It Slow...One Step at a Time*   For most people, healthy eating is a process. Little by little we make changes, we adjust, and then we get ready to change some more. For some, change means replacing a bag of potato chips at midnight with a healthier snack. For others, change means eating more broccoli. We all start from different places. What's important is to take it slow, one step at a time.

One

Fat . . . the Good, the Bad and the Ugly

Two Great Reasons to Eat Less Fat

Although healthy eating allows for a wide variety of foods, including those that are higher in fat, here are two great reasons to make lower-fat choices more often:

1. Saturated Fat = Artery-Lining Fat

Saturated fat is the type of fat found mostly in foods of animal origin, such as meats and dairy products. The widely acclaimed Seven Countries Study, involving more than 12,000 men in seven different countries, was one of the first to show its dangers. The study found that people who ate the most saturated fat were most likely to have high levels of cholesterol in their blood, and were more likely to suffer from heart disease. Other studies carried out around the world have confirmed the relationship between saturated fat intake and blood cholesterol levels.

Clear the Confusion
Healthy eating does not mean eating only low-fat foods. It means balancing your higher-fat choices with lower-fat choices. After all, it would be a crime not to enjoy a piece of cheese or chocolate on occasion. Eating is meant to be a pleasure.

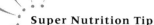

Super Nutrition Tip

With all the fuss about low-fat diets, don't forget that some fat is necessary. Fat provides a concentrated source of calories, especially important for young children, and certain fatty acids essential to proper growth and development of the brain and nervous system. And it helps carry essential vitamins such as A, D and E into the body, as well as assisting in their absorption.

The Top Ten Sources of Saturated Fat in the Canadian Diet
(in other words, the artery-lining kind)

1. Cheese
2. Butter
3. Milk
4. Cold cuts
5. Margarine
6. Ice cream
7. Ground beef
8. Bacon, sausage, wieners
9. Cooking/salad oils
10. Eggs

Please note:
1. Just because a food is on this list does not mean you shouldn't eat it. Milk and cheese are outstanding sources of calcium, while beef is an exceptional source of iron. The key message is to eat these foods in moderation and to choose the lower-fat options more often.
2. Most cooking/salad oils are low in saturated fat. They appear on the list because of the quantity of these products that we consume.

Source: Agriculture Canada Nutrient Assessment Program, based on data from the 1992 "Family Food Expenditure Survey" conducted by Statistics Canada

---

2. Too Much Fat Can Go to Your Hips

Fat has been called everything from a hip-liner to a waist-expander. This is because fat contains twice as many calories per gram as either protein or carbohydrate. As a result, foods that are high in fat are also high in calories. And although excess calories from any source, including protein and carbohydrate, can result in weight gain, your body is much more efficient at storing excess calories from fat than from other sources. Fat goes straight to the hips (and the waist and the legs and the butt).

Calories per gram

Carbohydrate = 4 calories

Protein = 4 calories

Fat = 9 calories

Translation: Eating more fat equals eating more calories.

News Flash: Fat Storage   Research from the University of Massachusetts Medical School suggests that if you consume 100 excess calories in the form of carbohydrate (foods like bread and pasta), 23 of those calories are used to convert the carbohydrate into fat and put it into storage. On the other hand, if you consume 100 excess calories from fat, a mere 3 calories are used to do the same thing. In other words, your body is much more efficient at storing excess calories from fat.

News Flash: Lower the Fat   Because fat is such a concentrated source of calories, it's a wise decision to limit your intake when trying to manage your waistline. Keep in mind, however, that because a food is low in fat it does not mean you can eat as much as you want without gaining weight. At the end of the day the total number of calories consumed is still important.

Read the Label
If a product is labelled "low in fat," it contains no more than 3 grams of fat per serving.

Reduce the Fat
A Montreal study has shown that people who assume that low-fat foods don't taste good are much less likely to make changes in their current diet. What's your attitude?

Six Questions People Frequently Ask about Fat

1. How Do Saturated Fats, Polyunsaturated Fats and Monounsaturated Fats Differ?

Fats and oils in our diet fall into three categories: polyunsaturated, monounsaturated and saturated, based on their chemical structure. All fats are made up of a combination, with one type predominating. For example, while olive oil is considered a monounsaturated fat, it contains some polyunsaturated fat and a small amount of saturated fat. Generally speaking, saturated fats are found in foods of animal origin. They are also used in the manufacturing of some processed foods. Polyunsaturated and monounsaturated fats are found primarily in foods of plant origin: fruits, vegetables, nuts, seeds, grains and the oils made from them. Remember: saturated fats raise blood cholesterol levels (they are artery-liners), while monounsaturated and polyunsaturated fats do just the opposite (they are heart-healthy fats). All fats are a concentrated source of calories (all are hip-liners).

Read the Label
If a product is labelled "light" or "lite," don't assume it's lower in fat or calories. These terms can apply to anything from colour to texture to taste to salt content. Take olive oil, for example. Many people buy "light" olive oil assuming it's lower in fat. In reality, the only thing "light" about it is the taste. It contains just as much fat and just as many calories as other oils. Your best bet is to read the fine print. The manufacturer should specify to what the term "light" refers.

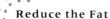

Reduce the Fat

With the exception of mayonnaise or mayonnaise-based sauces, condiments such as mustard, ketchup and relish are virtually fat-free.

Sources of Saturated Fat
(an artery-lining fat)

Meat (beef, pork, lamb), especially fatty cuts and ground meats

Processed meats such as sausages, hot dogs, side bacon and certain luncheon meats (bologna, liverwurst, salami)

Poultry, especially dark meat and poultry skin

Full-fat or partially fat dairy products (milk, cheese, butter, cream, ice cream)

Coconut and palm oil

Lard

Many processed foods (cookies, crackers, baked goods)

Chocolate

Sources of Polyunsaturated Fat
(a heart-healthy fat)

Vegetable oils (safflower, sunflower, corn, soybean)

Margarine

Fish

Nuts and seeds

Sources of Monounsaturated Fat
(a heart-healthy fat)

Vegetable oils (canola, olive, peanut)

Margarine

Nuts and seeds

Avocados

Olives

Read the Label

If the label says "Made with 100% vegetable oil," read the fine print on the ingredients list. Chances are the product has been made with hydrogenated vegetable oil, an artery-lining fat, as opposed to a heart-healthy fat.

Sources of Hydrogenated Fat
(an artery-lining fat)

Hard, stick margarines

Shortening

Many processed foods (cookies, crackers, snack foods, baked goods)

Many deep-fried foods (French fries, doughnuts)

---

2. What Is Hydrogenated Fat?

Hydrogenation (the adding of hydrogen) is a process used to make liquid oils more solid. The oils in margarine are partially hydrogenated to make a product that's spreadable. Hydrogenation also improves the shelf life and stability of many baked goods and processed foods. Now for the bad news. Hydrogenation changes a healthy, unsaturated fat into one that acts like an unhealthy, saturated one (the technical term for these fats is trans fatty acids). There are three things you can do to limit your intake of hydrogenated fats. First, choose soft tub margarines rather than hard stick margarines (the more solid the margarine, the more hydrogenated the product). Second, because it's almost impossible to avoid the hydrogenated fat in baked goods and processed foods, choose the lower-fat products more often. Last but not least, limit your intake of deep-fried fatty foods like French fries. Most are cooked in hydrogenated vegetable oils.

3. Is Margarine Better Than Butter?

Fact: butter contains artery-lining saturated fat. Fact: margarine contains artery-lining hydrogenated fat. Which one is better? First, whether you choose margarine or butter, the most important message is simply to use less of it. Second, a good soft tub margarine (non-hydrogenated and low in saturated fat) such as Becel or President's Choice 7 Reasons Margarine contains significantly less artery-lining fat than butter. Third, even better than butter or margarine are the "light" margarines such as Becel Light, with 50% less fat and fewer calories.

4. Should I Avoid Foods with Cholesterol?

Do you suffer from cholesterolphobia, the fear of foods containing cholesterol? If so, your fear may be unwarranted. For many people, cholesterol in the diet has little effect on the levels of cholesterol in the blood. When it comes to heart health the main offenders are the saturated and hydrogenated fats. In any case, since saturated fats and cholesterol are found in many of the same foods, when you limit your intake of saturated fat (which is definitely a good thing), you automatically limit your intake of cholesterol as well. (See section on eggs on p.53 for more information)

5. What Are "Good" Cholesterol and "Bad" Cholesterol?

First of all, the terms "good" and "bad" cholesterol have nothing (absolutely nothing!) to do with the cholesterol in food. They describe the cholesterol in your blood. Cholesterol in your blood is found primarily in one of two forms – HDL or "good" cholesterol and LDL or "bad" cholesterol. LDL is responsible for the accumulation of plaque (thick, yellow cholesterol deposits) on the artery wall. HDL, on the other hand, is responsible for removing cholesterol from your blood.

Clear the Confusion
Although the sign at the fast-food outlet says "We use only 100% vegetable oil," chances are it is hydrogenated vegetable oil they are talking about. Translation: deep-fried foods equal artery-lining foods.

Clear the Confusion
Many people mistakenly believe that margarine contains less fat and fewer calories than butter. They are actually exactly the same. The only difference is the type of fat they contain. Most soft tub margarines contain less artery-lining fats than butter.

Sources of Cholesterol

Eggs
Meat, especially organ meats (liver, kidney)
Processed meats (sausages, some luncheon meats, hot dogs)
Full-fat dairy products (cheese, butter, cream, ice cream)
Shellfish (crab, lobster, shrimp)

Read the Label

Don't be duped by labels that shout "No cholesterol" or "Cholesterol-free." Many foods that happily proclaim their cholesterol-free status–foods like potato chips or vegetable oils–never contained any cholesterol in the first place. How could they? Cholesterol is found only in foods of animal origin. What's more, many of these foods are very high in fat. When reading labels, focus on how much fat a product contains, not on cholesterol.

Reduce the Fat

Get a good nonstick pan and use a vegetable oil spray instead of butter or margarine for cooking.

Ideally, you want high levels of HDL and low levels of LDL. Many factors can influence your levels of HDL and LDL. For example, a diet high in saturated fat results in higher levels of LDL or "bad" cholesterol.

6. Is Olive Oil the Best Kind of Oil?

The benefits of the Mediterranean diet, which includes liberal amounts of olive oil, have been much touted lately. As a result, the sales of olive oil have skyrocketed. Does olive oil promote optimal health? Here are five things you should know:

1. Fat of any kind should be consumed in moderation, especially when you consider how concentrated it is when it comes to calories.

2. People should be more concerned about reducing saturated fat and total fat overall than about which type of oil to buy.

3. All oils, with the exception of coconut and palm oil, are considered heart-healthy.

4. Based on studies, such as those reviewing the benefits of the Mediterranean diet, some health experts recommend monounsaturated fats like olive oil and canola oil over polyunsaturated fats like corn oil and sunflower oil. Current Canadian guidelines, however, do not recommend the use of one over the other.

5. Some researchers believe that canola oil, because of the omega-3 fats it contains, may provide some additional benefits in terms of heart health.

Bottom line: cutting back on total fats and using a variety of different unsaturated fats is probably the wisest decision overall.

News Flash: Chocolate Lovers' Relief While too much chocolate can wreak havoc on your waistline, it may be fine for your heart. Chocolate contains mostly stearic acid, a type of saturated fat that is believed to be less harmful than most other saturated fats.

How Much Fat?

The 30% Guideline

The average woman needs about 1,900 calories a day, while the average man needs about 2,700 calories. According to current guidelines, fat should provide no more than 30% of total daily calories. Translated (at 9 calories per gram of fat) this means that women should consume no more than about 65 grams of fat per day, and men should limit their intake to 90 grams. The best way to achieve this is by eating lean meats, low-fat dairy products, and lots of fruits, vegetables and whole grains; and by going easy on high-fat foods like butter, margarine and cooking oils. Use the fat graphs in this book to get a rough estimate of your daily fat gram intake.

It Doesn't Have to Be an All-or-Nothing Affair

Many people are under the impression that the only way to limit your fat intake to 30% of calories is to eat only foods that contain 30% fat or less. By this rule, however, foods like peanut butter, cheese, butter and margarine would all be strictly off limits. Most people would prefer to cut back on the use of these products rather than say goodbye to them altogether. The best way to do this is to balance your higher-fat choices with some lower-fat choices. For example, to balance the fat in a peanut butter sandwich, eat it with lower fat choices like carrot sticks, an apple and a glass of skim milk.

What about Kids?

From the age of two until the time when a child reaches his or her full height (usually mid to late teens) there should be a gradual transition from the high-fat diet of infancy to a diet that includes no more than

---

Daily Fat Gram Quota

Women – 65 grams
Men – 90 grams

Reduce the Fat
People report that one of the most enjoyable changes when switching to a low-fat diet is eating more fruits and vegetables.

Read the Label
Balance out your higher-fat choices with lower-fat choices. If the percentage of calories coming from fat is not listed on the label, the following calculation can be used to determine the percentage:

(Grams of fat x 9) ÷ by total calories x 100 = % of calories from fat

For example, 1 SnackWell Chocolate Sandwich Cookie contains 54 calories and 1.0 gram of fat. The equation looks like this: (1 x 9) ÷ 54 x 100 = 17% of calories from fat.

Read the Label

To check at a glance whether 30% or less of the calories in a product are in the form of fat, keep this in mind: for every 100 calories of food, there should be no more than 3 grams of fat. For example, if a product contains 200 calories, it should contain no more than 6 grams of fat.

Reduce the Fat

Butter, margarine, mayonnaise, salad dressings and cooking oils are very high in fat (most are 100% fat). Even small changes in your consumption of these foods can reduce your fat intake significantly.

30% of energy as fat. Fat should never be restricted in the diet of children prior to the age of two. Breast milk contains over 50% of its calories in the form of fat for a good reason. Babies have very high calorie needs relative to their tiny size, and fat provides a concentrated source of the calories and essential fats necessary for proper growth and development. (For more information on the fat requirements of children and adolescents, see p.158.)

Where Is It Coming From?

The majority of fat in the Canadian diet comes primarily from four sources: fats and oils added to other foods, baked goods, fatty meats, and high-fat dairy products. Throughout the rest of this book you'll find lots of fat-reducing ideas for decreasing the amount of fat from these and other sources.

The Top Ten Sources of Fat in the Canadian Diet
Foods Containing All Types of Fat

1. Butter/margarine
2. Cooking oils/salad dressings/mayonnaise
3. Baked goods (breads, cakes, cookies, pies)
4. Cold cuts
5. Cheese
6. Fresh beef (including ground beef)
7. Milk
8. Nuts and peanut butter
9. Bacon, sausages, wieners
10. Ice cream

Source: Agriculture Canada Nutrient Assessment Program, based on data from the 1992 "Family Food Expenditure Survey" conducted by Statistics Canada.

The Added Fats and Oils Story

Based on a 15 mL (1 tbsp) serving size

	Grams of fat
Oil	14
Butter	12
Margarine	12
Mayonnaise	11
Salad Dressing	8

Please note: One serving of the average salad contains about 3 to 5 tablespoons (45 mL–75 mL) of dressing.

In a Nutshell...

Eat less fat, especially the artery-lining saturated and hydrogenated fats. If you're like most Canadians, butter, margarine, mayonnaise, salad dressings and cooking oils contribute more fat to your diet than any other foods. Fatty cuts of meat, many processed meats and full-fat dairy products are the main contributors of saturated fat. All fats contain concentrated amounts of calories and can be damaging to the waistline.

Two

Eat Fruits & Vegetables by the Truckload

The Number One Reason to Eat Fruits and Vegetables by the Truckload

(This is the part of the book where I want to jump up and down and wave my arms madly in the air just to make sure you're paying attention.)

Prescription for Super Health

Do you want a simple prescription for good health? Eat fruits and vegetables – lots of them. Research study after research study after research study (more than 200 studies to date), from the Mediterranean to the Far East, has come to the same conclusion: people who eat lots of fruits and vegetables can reduce their risk of both heart disease and cancer by as much as 50%. Read on to find out why.

Fruit and Vegetable Trivia
On any given day your average supermarket has more than 225 different fruits and vegetables for sale.

Four Things That Make Fruits and Vegetables Incredible

1. Vitamin C, Folic Acid, Fibre and More

On average, Canadians get 86% of their vitamin C, over 44% of their vitamin A (mostly in the form of beta-carotene), and almost 40% of their folic acid and fibre from fruits and vegetables. That's significant – especially when you consider that each of these nutrients has been identified as a key player in the prevention of disease. Magnesium, copper and potassium, other essential nutrients for good health, are also found in good supply in fruits and vegetables.

2. They Are Virtually Fat-Free

You could search the entire produce department, aisle by aisle, top to bottom, and be hard pressed to find a single fat gram anywhere. That's right. With the exception of avocados, coconuts and olives, fruits and vegetables are virtually fat-free. Nutritious, delicious and fat-free: it doesn't get any better than that.

Reduce the Fat

Although eggplant itself contains hardly any fat, it absorbs fat easily. When fried, 1 serving can absorb 83 grams of fat (more than 700 calories) in just 70 seconds–four times as much as an equal portion of potatoes. If you love eggplant, steam, bake, or grill it.

The Fruit and Vegetable Story

	Grams of fat
Avocado, 1/2	15.0
Coconut, shredded (125 mL/1/2 cup)	17.0
Olives, 5 large green	5.0
Banana, 1	.6
Apple, 1	.5
Carrot, 1	.2
Spinach (250 mL/1 cup)	.2

Please note: With the exception of avocados, coconuts and olives, all fruits and vegetables contain less than 1 gram of fat per serving. And the fat found in olives and avocados is primarily the monounsaturated, heart-healthy kind.

3. Fruits and Vegetables Contain Antioxidants

Special kinds of vitamins, called antioxidants, have been referred to as everything from "mother nature's white knights" to "mighty warriors against disease." Research indicates they play an important role in the prevention of disease, particularly heart disease, cancer and cataracts.

Here's how they work: when an apple is sliced, oxygen in the air reacts with the cut surface to turn it brown. We call this process oxidation. If, however, the apple slices are dipped in orange or lemon juice, the slices stay white much longer. The vitamin C in the juice acts as an antioxidant. It prevents the oxygen from combining with the apple. The same thing happens in our bodies. When our bodies use oxygen, by-products called "free radicals" are produced. Free radicals are also produced in our bodies when we are exposed to cigarette smoke or pollution. Just as the oxygen in the air can damage the surface of the sliced apple, free radicals in our bodies can harm our cells. They increase our risk of disease by making our artery walls more prone to the build-up of cholesterol and by initiating or enhancing cancer development. The good news is that by consuming a diet rich in antioxidants, like vitamin C, vitamin E and beta-carotene, we help prevent the damage caused by free radicals and thereby reduce our risk of disease. Dark green and orange fruits and vegetables are the richest sources of antioxidants in our diets, particularly for vitamin C and beta-carotene. (For information on antioxidant supplements, see p.140.)

Reduce the Fat
Instead of drowning your vegetables in butter, drizzle them with fresh lemon juice, followed by a sprinkle of Parmesan cheese.

> **News Flash: Vegetables of the Future** Scientists are experimenting with "vegetable leather," a soft, pliable green sheet similar to fruit roll-ups but made of vegetables. The world of snacking may never be the same.

4. Fruits and Vegetables Contain Phytochemicals

Fruits and vegetables contain hundreds, perhaps thousands, of phytochemicals. Phytochemicals are simply chemicals found in plants. Although they're not nutrients like vitamins and minerals, researchers believe that many phytochemicals help prevent cancer and heart disease in one of three ways. As antioxidants, they put a stop to cell-damaging free radicals. As blocking agents, they prevent the activation of carcinogens (things that cause cancer). As suppressing agents, they stop the cancer process in cells previously exposed to carcinogens. Some of the fruits and vegetables that have been identified as containing beneficial phytochemicals are broccoli, cabbage, citrus fruits, apples, grapes, berries (strawberries, raspberries, blueberries), and allium vegetables like onions, leeks and garlic.

Four Things to Consider When Choosing Fruits and Vegetables

1. The Dark Green and Orange Rule

Super Nutrition Tip
Romaine lettuce has four times as much vitamin C and beta-carotene, and twice as much folic acid, as iceberg lettuce.

Generally speaking, the more vibrant and intense the colour of a fruit or vegetable, the greater its nutritional value. More specifically, dark green and orange fruits and vegetables offer the greatest bang for your nutritional buck. For example, spinach and romaine are much richer in nutrients than iceberg lettuce. Carrots are far more nutritious than celery. Cantaloupes are more nutritious than honeydew melons. Mangoes are more nutritious than apples. Keep in mind that it is the colour of the flesh, not the skin, of the fruit or vegetable that is usually the most meaningful. Cucumbers, although dark green on the outside, are very pale on the inside and thus don't rank as nutritional all-stars.

2. The Splendiferous Cruciferous

Cruciferous vegetables are generating a lot of excitement these days because of their rich nutrient content, as well as the beneficial phyto-chemicals they contain. Broccoli, which contains the phytochemical sulforaphane, has often been singled out in this group (the King of Cruciferous Vegetables).

3. The Top Ten

This "Top Ten" list of fruits and vegetables takes into account both the Dark Green and Orange Rule and the Splendiferous Cruciferous factor, and provides you with the "Best of the Best" from an overall nutritional standpoint.

Cruciferous Vegetables All-Star List	
Bok Choy	Kale
Broccoli	Kohlrabi
Brussels sprouts	Mustard greens
Cabbage	Rutabagas
Cauliflower	Turnip roots and greens
Collards	

The Top Ten
(In alphabetical order for your viewing pleasure)

1. Broccoli (and all its cruciferous relatives)
2. Cantaloupe
3. Carrots
4. Mangoes (papayas are also excellent)
5. Oranges (and other citrus fruits like tangerines and grapefruits)
6. Red peppers (green peppers are also great)
7. Spinach (and other dark leafy greens like kale and swiss chard)
8. Strawberries (and other berries like raspberries and blueberries)
9. Sweet potatoes (potatoes, squash and pumpkin are also excellent)
10. Tomatoes

Cooking Tip
To avoid losing nutrients, cook vegetables in a minimal amount of water and only until they reach the "tender but crisp" stage.

4. Eat at Least Five a Day for Better Health

To optimize the nutritional benefits and reduce your risk of disease, health experts recommend a minimum of 5 servings of fruits and vegetables each day. (Canada's Food Guide to Healthy Eating recommends 5 to 10 servings per day, with the higher number of servings intended for people with higher calorie needs.) This 5-a-day minimum may seem overwhelming, but once you understand what is meant by 1 serving, you'll see that meeting your quota is no big deal.

One Serving Is Equal to:

1 medium-size fruit or vegetable (apple, orange, banana, potato, carrot)

125 mL ($^1/_2$ cup) of any fresh, frozen or canned fruit or vegetable

250 mL (1 cup) of salad

125 mL ($^1/_2$ cup) of any fruit or vegetable juice

50 mL ($^1/_4$ cup) of dried fruit

Eighteen Great Tips for Adding More Fruits and Vegetables to Your Life

When asked why they don't eat more fruits and vegetables, people usually say they are inconvenient, or time-consuming, or just plain boring. Fruits and vegetables don't have to be any of these things. Here are 18 great tips to up your intake of these super-healthy foods.

1. Think Fruit or Veg

Every time you get hungry and feel like munching on something, think fruit or veg. Before you reach for any other food, ask yourself, "What fruit or vegetable could I munch on right now ?" Practise this habit for one month and you'll be amazed how easy it is to up your intake of the good stuff.

Tomato Trivia

The tomato is botanically a fruit, but a decision by the U.S. Supreme Court, way back in 1893, declared it legally a vegetable.

2. Eliminate the Competition

Imagine this scenario. You're sitting at a desk. In the right-hand drawer is a bright red juicy apple. In your left-hand drawer is a melt-in-your-mouth milk chocolate and hazelnut bar. Which one will you eat first? If you are like most people (me included), the apple doesn't stand a chance. If, however, you eliminate the competition – the chocolate bar – the apple's appeal increases tenfold, especially at about four in the afternoon when hunger often strikes. Keep the tempting competition out of reach – at work and at home – and you'll find healthy eating much easier.

Keep It Fresh

Don't keep fruits and vegetables in the same drawer of your fridge. Most fruits give off ethylene, a harmless natural gas that causes veggies to spoil more quickly.

3. In Sight, in Mind

You've heard the phrase "out of sight, out of mind." Well, the reverse is also true. If you have plenty of fruits and vegetables "in sight," they are much more likely to also be "in mind." For example, kids are much more likely to grab a piece of fruit for a snack when it's in view and within easy reach. Similarly, if you keep a bowl of fruit handy at work, you'll be much more likely to indulge (as will all your co-workers).

4. The Never-Skip-a-Meal Deal

Meeting your 5-a-day quota is easy when you eat fruits or vegetables with every meal. For example, have a small glass of juice with your breakfast, a piece of fruit with your morning snack, a small salad or a few carrot sticks with your lunch and a couple of vegetables or a salad with your dinner. It's that easy.

5. Sandwich It

Sandwiches are a great place to "veg out." Next time you make or buy a sandwich, pile on the veggies. Sliced tomatoes, cucumbers, dark green leafy lettuce and strips of green pepper add not only crunch, but pizzazz. When you really want to go to town, add a tangy coleslaw mixture to your sandwich (great with chicken). Simply mix shredded cabbage with a creamy low-fat salad dressing.

6. Focus on Foods You Enjoy

Here's a simple concept – focus on foods you enjoy. Pick foods you currently enjoy and add more fruits or vegetables to them. Let's take lasagna. Some of the best lasagnas I've tasted were layered with broccoli, carrots, spinach and more. The same can be done with your favourite chili, spaghetti sauce, casserole or rice dish. As for fruit, add

Super Nutrition Tip
In a recent study, the microwave came out on top for preserving the nutrients in cooked vegetables.

Keep It Fresh
Bags designed specifically for storing vegetables in your home, such as Ziploc Vegetable Bags, really do work. The tiny vents in each bag slow down spoilage by holding in just the right amount of moisture.

Taste Tip
If you brown-bag your lunch and love tomatoes, here's a tip for you. Rather than adding sliced tomatoes to your sandwich in the morning and having a soggy sandwich by noon, pack the tomato slices in a separate container and add them only when you're ready to take your first bite.

Taste Tip
A great way to enhance the taste of your vegetables is with a touch of sugar. Glazed carrots happen to be one of my favourites. And squash just wouldn't be the same without a drizzle of maple syrup, a dab of butter or margarine and a pinch of nutmeg.

some to your cereal, pancake or muffin mix. And remember, every little bite helps and a whole bunch of little bites adds up to a whole lot of fruits and vegetables.

7. Dare to Be Different

Go out on a limb, live on the edge, dare to be different, expand your horizons. I'm talking mangoes, kiwis, tangerines, papayas, kale, swiss chard – and the list goes on. Never before have Canadians had access to such a wide selection of fruits and vegetables. An apple is refreshing, but a mango is divinely delicious (and so nutritious too). Make a pact with yourself to buy at least one daringly different fruit or vegetable to savour each week.

8. Don't Leave Home without Them

Keep portable fruits like apples and bananas with you at all times – in your car, in your briefcase, at your desk. Your fruit consumption will escalate by leaps and bounds.

9. Soup's On

Soup is the perfect home for vegetables of all shapes, kinds and sizes. A warm soup in winter is comfort food at its best. A chilled soup in summer is cool and refreshing. From minestrone to gazpacho, the options are endless.

10. Let's Get Green, without the Grease

The most popular item ordered at restaurants, next to French fries, is salad. Salads are a wonderful way to up your vegetable intake, as long as you go easy on the high-fat dressings and pick the more nutritious greens, like spinach or romaine, more often.

11. It's More Than Rabbit Food

Everybody's heard the "apple a day" advice. Well, what about a carrot a day? Picture this...you just got home, you've had a long day at work, you're tired and hungry. Stop right there. Before you make yourself some dinner, before you grab a snack out of the cupboard, peel yourself one carrot (or just scrub it and leave the peel on for extra fibre) and eat it. One lone carrot is all I'm asking. This "carrot-a-day" ritual could have a significant effect on your health. How significant? In a recent study involving over 87,000 females, those who consumed 5 or more servings of carrots a week had a significantly lower stroke risk compared with women who ate them no more than once a month. So, get your friends, your family and your relatives into the act. Keep your fridge well stocked. And eat those carrots. (If you want to eat an apple a day too, great!)

Reduce the Fat
Salad dressing continues to be one of the top sources of fat in the Canadian diet. When making salad dressing, cut down on fat by replacing some of the oil with water, stock, wine, buttermilk, or low-fat yogurt. Flavoured vinegars, like raspberry or balsamic, also allow you to use less oil without losing out on taste.

12. Let's Get Juiced

If you can't eat 'em, juice 'em. The next best thing to whole fruits and vegetables is their juice. Juice provides a concentrated liquid hit of great nutrition, as long as you keep three things in mind. First, all the wonderful fibre found in fruits and vegetables is removed during the juicing process. Second, fruit juice is a fairly concentrated source of calories, while most vegetable juices are high in salt. Third, too much fruit juice can interfere with the healthy appetites of young children. Best advice: enjoy your juice, but eat most of your fruits and vegetables whole.

Super Nutrition Tip
Here is a list of fruit juices ranked from most to least nutritious: Orange, grapefruit, prune, pineapple, cranberry, grape, apple, pear.

Read the Label
Anything called fruit "drink," "beverage," "punch," "-ade," or "cocktail" usually contains very little fruit juice–the rest being water and sugar.

News Flash: Cranberry Juice   Scientists have confirmed that cranberry juice contains a substance that prevents bladder infections by keeping bacteria from latching onto the walls of the urinary tract.

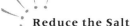

Reduce the Salt
The main disadvantage of canned vegetables compared to either fresh or frozen is the added salt they often contain.

Reduce the Fat
Here's how to stir-fry with as little fat as possible:
Use a nonstick pan and little if any fat during cooking. Instead of cooking oil, use 1/4 cup (50 mL) water, or, for extra flavour, chicken or vegetable broth, for every 1 cup (250 mL) of cut vegetables. Boil the liquid alone first, then lower the heat to medium and add the vegetables, stirring until tender-crisp. Like magic, vegetables cooked to perfection, with no added fat.

13. Canned and Frozen Fruits and Veggies

Who said that canned or frozen fruits and vegetables are not high-quality nutritional choices? On the contrary, these fruits and vegetables are harvested at the peak of ripeness, then prepared for canning or freezing within hours of being picked. This speed guarantees not only great taste but excellent nutritional quality as well. What's more, much of the fresh produce available during the winter months has lost nutrients during travelling time and storage. And for convenience, canned and frozen goods can't be beat.

14. Grill It

Grilling, especially on a barbecue, is a delicious, easy way to cook fresh vegetables. The dry heat helps to retain vitamins while adding that distinctive smoked flavour. Basting vegetables as they cook helps them remain tender and moist while giving them a caramelized crust. For a quick marinade use low-fat salad dressing.

15. Let's Get Dipping

Vegetables and dip. Is there a more splendid combination? Even kids who faint at the sight of anything green will consume a tray full of veggies and dip in seconds. If you think that veggies and dip are too time-consuming, buy precut veggies and dip in a low-fat salad dressing. And the next time you go to a party and you see a huge tray of fresh-cut veggies, indulge, enjoy, eat up (someone has done all that peeling and chopping for you).

16. I Love Dessert

Whether it's fresh berries served over frozen yogurt, or applesauce heated with cinnamon and brown sugar, fruit is a great way to satisfy our craving for something sweet at the end of a meal. (See the section on desserts for more great ideas.)

17. Double Up

Still wondering how to squeeze those 5 to 10 servings into your diet? Why not try doubling up. If you normally have one scoop of mashed potatoes, have two. If you normally have one spoonful of peas, take an extra spoonful. If you normally have half a banana with your cereal, have a whole banana. It doesn't get any simpler than that.

18. Come to Grips with the Chocolate Thing

Here it is. Chocolate tastes better than carrot sticks – to most people anyway. Despite that, at some point, you have to make a conscious decision to eat more fruits and vegetables. Considering the protective shield of antioxidants, phytochemicals and essential nutrients they contain, it's a wise investment in your health.

A Word about Pesticides

If, like the majority of Canadians, you are concerned about chemical residues in or on food, here are four things you should know:

1. Health Canada is responsible for determining a level of pesticide residues that is safe not only for the general public, but also for infants, children and pregnant women. Although some imported produce may be more likely to contain pesticide residues, it is required to meet the same standards.
2. Scientists today can measure even the smallest amounts of pesticide residues, and tests indicate that Canada's food supply is almost completely free of pesticide residues.
3. The American Medical Association's Council on Scientific Affairs recently examined all the scientific evidence to date related to cancer and pesticides. Their conclusion: "The levels of synthetic

pesticide residues in food seem so low as to be of no consequence whatever."

4. Based on a report by the American Institute of Food Technologists' Expert Panel on Food Safety, many scientists do not consider organic produce (grown without pesticides) either safer or more healthful than produce grown using conventional methods. In other words, the need to buy organic produce is unwarranted.

In addition, farmers are rethinking traditional methods of crop protection. Integrated pest management (IPM) is one such example. Pesticides are used only when nonchemical alternatives (such as crop rotation or the introduction of beneficial insects to eat more harmful ones) won't work.

In the meantime, to minimize your risk from pesticides (however small that risk may be), you can do four things. First, wash thoroughly all fresh produce before you eat it (the use of soap or detergent is not recommended). Second, discard the outer leaves of leafy vegetables like lettuce and cabbage. Third, remove the peel from those fruits or vegetables that have an obvious wax-like coating, like apples and cucumbers. Fourth, certain fruits such as strawberries, cherries and grapes may be more likely to contain pesticide residues and should be washed especially well. Most importantly, relax and enjoy the truly remarkable benefits that come with eating fruits and vegetables.

In a Nutshell...

Eating more fruits and vegetables can significantly reduce your risk of developing both heart disease and cancer. Fruits and vegetables are low in fat and are an important source of many essential nutrients, including vitamin C, vitamin A, folic acid and fibre. They contain antioxidants and phytochemicals, which are thought to play a key role in the prevention of disease. Eat 5 to 10 servings each day.

Three

Be a Whole-Grain, High-Fibre Feaster

Top Three Reasons to Enjoy the Greatness of Grains (like breads, cereals, rice and pasta)

People from far and wide listen with eager anticipation to reports about the virtues of life in the Mediterranean. Here is a place known for its lower rates of heart disease and cancer, a place where red wine and olive oil flow freely, and where fruits and vegetables are consumed in abundance. Yet there is another aspect of life in the Mediterranean that's equally fascinating, although much less talked about. It's the core, the foundation, the very heart of the diet. It's the food around which every meal revolves – grains. The entire grain family takes centre stage in this healthful diet – breads, rice, pastas and more. Not surprisingly, nutrition experts recommend grain products as the cornerstone of healthy eating for these three reasons:

1. Carbohydrates, Iron, Trace Minerals and More

Grains are rich in carbohydrates, the primary source of fuel for our bodies. Health Canada recommends we get most (55%) of our daily calories from carbohydrates. Grains help us meet our need for B vitamins (especially thiamin and folic acid) and iron. A lack of iron can leave us feeling tired and decrease our resistance to infections. Grains – with the emphasis on whole grains – contain vitamin E, which is important for heart health. Whole grains also provide trace minerals – like zinc, selenium, copper, manganese, chromium and magnesium – that are often in short supply in our diets. Last but not least, grains are gaining attention for the beneficial plant compounds (phytochemicals) they contain and their potential to reduce the risk of heart disease and cancer.

> **News Flash: Folic Acid**   In both Canada and the United States folic acid is now added to grain products such as flour and pasta in reponse to evidence that women who get adequate amounts of folic acid (.4 mg/day) are less likely to have babies with certain birth defects of the brain and spinal cord (neural tube defects). Folic acid may also play an important role in the prevention of heart disease.

2. Grains Are Low in Fat

Contrary to popular belief, grains are not fattening. Most grain products – like breads, cereals, rice and pasta – contain a mere 1 to 2 grams of fat per serving. The fats that are naturally present in these foods are primarily the heart-healthy unsaturated kind. The only problem with grains is not the grains themselves, but the high-fat spreads (like butter or margarine) and sauces (like Alfredo) that often accompany them.

The Grain Story
(without added spreads or sauces)

Grain products are low in fat. It's what you add to them that causes their fat content to escalate.

	Grams of fat
Rice (250 mL/1 cup)	1.0
Bread (1 slice)	1.0
Pasta (250 mL/1 cup)	1.0
Tortilla (1)	1.0
Cereal (small bowl)	1.0

3. Fibre All-Stars

Without doubt, one of the greatest contributions made by whole grains is fibre. Fibre is largely plant-cell material that resists digestion. It moves unaltered through the stomach and small intestine and into the colon. There are two types of fibre – soluble and insoluble. Soluble fibre is most important for heart health and blood sugar control. Insoluble fibre is most significant for preventing constipation, as well as reducing the risk of certain cancers. Both kinds of fibre are important for weight control. Eating a variety of whole grains, fruits, vegetables and beans is the best way to optimize your fibre intake.

Five Fabulous Things about Fibre

1. Fibre Keeps Things "Moving Along"

Insoluble fibre, which is found in wheat bran and some fruits and vegetables, is well known for its ability to prevent or relieve constipation. By increasing stool bulk (it absorbs many times its weight in water) fibre promotes more efficient elimination and also reduces the incidence of hemorrhoids and diverticular disease (pouches or pockets that form in the wall of the colon). All whole wheat products, including breads and cereals, are a good source of wheat bran. Psyllium, a soluble fibre, is also known for its strong laxative effect.

2. Cancer Prevention

Based on data from 12 different countries, it appears that our risk of colon cancer could be reduced by more than 30% by eating more high-fibre foods. Researchers believe that by speeding the movement of digested food through the intestines, insoluble fibre reduces the amount of time the colon is exposed to cancer-promoting substances. Insoluble fibre may also reduce the risk of breast cancer by decreasing

Clear the Confusion
Because bread is already so low in fat, most "diet" or "light" breads are just thinner, smaller slices of the same stuff you normally eat.

Hydration Tip
Because fibre attracts water to your intestines, a high-fibre diet should be complemented by a high fluid intake.

Super Nutrition Tip
Flaxseed and flaxseed oil (also called linseed oil) may help ward off both heart disease and cancer. Add whole or ground flaxseed, available at health food stores and some supermarkets, to muffin recipes or sprinkle it on your cereal. In recipes for muffins or other baked goods, replace 30% to 50% of the all-purpose flour with ground flaxseed.

the levels of circulating hormones, such as estrogen, that are involved in its development.

3. Heart Protector

A study involving 43,000 male health professionals indicates that a high-fibre diet can reduce the risk of heart disease by more than 35%. While both types of fibre may be important, soluble fibre is known for its ability to reduce the amount of cholesterol in our blood. The best grain sources of soluble fibre are foods that contain oat bran (found in oatmeal) or psyllium (found in cereals like Bran Buds). Fruits, vegetables and beans are also important sources of soluble fibre.

4. Weight Control

Studies show that overweight individuals often eat significantly less fibre than healthy-weight individuals. Researchers believe that fibre helps to control weight by regulating the appetite. When you eat more fibre, you feel more satisfied and eat less of other foods. In addition, most high-fibre foods are low in calories and fat. So don't cut the bread out of your diet – just make sure it's whole grain, and keep the butter to a minimum.

5. Blood Sugar Control

Soluble fibre may help people with diabetes control their blood sugar levels by slowing the absorption of glucose (sugar) from carbohydrates.

Super Nutrition Tip

While oat bran may be good for the heart, it's not without competition. New on the horizon is psyllium, a natural grain grown primarily in India, that has eight times as much soluble fibre (the kind that helps lower blood cholesterol levels) as oat bran.

Fibre Source Recap

Best Sources of Soluble Fibre
(lowers blood cholesterol levels)

    Oat bran

    Oatmeal

    Psyllium (in cereals like Bran Buds)

    Legumes (dried beans, peas and
      lentils)

    Pectin rich fruits (apples, strawber-
      ries, citrus fruits)

    Flaxseed

Best Sources of Insoluble Fibre
(prevents constipation and reduces risk
of some cancers)

    Wheat bran

    Whole wheat breads and cereals

    Wheat bran cereals

    Fruits and vegetables (including the
      skins and seeds when practical)

Super Nutrition Tip

If you're currently a low-fibre eater and are convinced it's now time to become a high-fibre feaster, please restrain your enthusiasm. This unbridled zeal may leave you bloated and gassy. Instead, up your intake over the period of a few weeks to give your body time to adjust.

Have You Met Your Fibre Quota Today?

Most health professionals recommend an intake of 25 to 35 grams of fibre every day. Recent surveys indicate, however, that most Canadians consume about 15 grams per day, or about half of the recommended daily intake.

Read the Label

If the label says...	The food contains...
Source of dietary fibre	At least 2 grams of fibre per serving
High source of dietary fibre	At least 4 grams of fibre per serving
Very high source of dietary fibre	At least 6 grams of fibre per serving

The Quickie Method for Calculating Your Daily Fibre Intake

Write down everything you eat for one day and then use this list to estimate your daily fibre intake.

	Grams of fibre
Slice of whole grain bread*	2
Bowl of cereal**	2
Scoop of brown rice	2
Small plate of pasta	2
Piece of fruit	2
Serving of vegetables	2
Handful of nuts	2
Small serving of beans	5

  * *If the bread and rice are not whole grain, for example, whole wheat bread or brown rice, count only 1 gram of fibre per serving.*

  ** *This is a rough estimate only. Many cereals, for example, contain more than 2 grams of fibre, while others contain less.*

News Flash: Fibre for Kids   Children over the age of three can gradually add more fibre to their diet by the "age-plus-5" formula. An amount equal to, or greater than, their age, plus 5, is about the amount of fibre children need each day. For example, a 3-year-old should consume about 8 grams of fibre per day, while a 10-year-old should consume about 15 grams.

Top Ten Things You Should Know about Grains

1. Eat Five to Twelve Servings Each Day

Super Nutrition Tip
A sprinkle of wheat bran on cereal, pancakes or muffins is a great way to increase the fibre content of those foods.

Canada's Food Guide to Healthy Eating recommends 5 to12 servings of grain products each day. Individuals with lower calorie needs, such as young children, can choose the minimum number of servings, while those with higher calorie needs, such as an active male teenager, can choose the higher number of servings. Most of us can choose servings somewhere in between.

One Serving Equals:
1 slice of bread
175 mL ($^3/_4$ cup) of hot cereal
30 g of cold cereal (most cereal box labels will tell you exactly what 30 g is equal to, for example, 30 g of Cheerios = 325 mL or $1^1/_3$ cups)
$^1/_2$ bagel
$^1/_2$ pita bread
$^1/_2$ hamburger bun
125 mL ($^1/_2$ cup) rice
125 mL ($^1/_2$ cup) pasta

Please note: Few people sit down to just half a cup of pasta at one meal; more likely, their plate of spaghetti represents 3 or 4 servings of grain products. Few people eat just half a bagel. Therefore, when eating a whole bagel be sure to count it as 2 servings (a jumbo-size bagel counts as four servings). This same logic applies throughout the grain serving checklist.

2. Make It "Whole" Grain

What exactly is meant by "whole grain"? All grain kernels are made up of three main parts – the bran, the germ and the endosperm. The bran, or outer covering, supplies some B vitamins and most of the minerals and fibre. The germ, located at the base of the kernel, also supplies B vitamins, along with most of the vitamin E. The endosperm, or inner core, is composed primarily of starch (carbohydrate) and some protein. Manufacturers of refined products, such as white bread or white rice, use only the endosperm and discard the bran and germ along with most of the fibre and much of the nutrition. To enrich their products, manufacturers replace some of the nutrients lost during processing – some of the B vitamins (thiamin, riboflavin, niacin, folic acid) and iron. In most cases, what is not replaced is the fibre, the vitamin E and most of the trace minerals, nutrients that are essential to good health and often in short supply in our diets.

Bottom line: whole grain products (like whole wheat bread, whole wheat pasta and brown rice) contain the nutrient-rich, fibre-rich bran and germ, and are much more nutritious than their refined, endosperm-only counterparts.

3. Perfect Breads

Although 12-grain bread may sound like the ultimate high-fibre choice, these breads frequently contain mostly white flour with just a sprinkling of 11 other grains. Similarly, breads like pumpernickel, oatmeal and rye often contain white flour as the primary ingredient. Look for those breads that list whole grains, like whole wheat flour, first on the ingredient list (ingredients are always listed in the order of the amount used). Generally speaking, nothing beats the fibre and nutrition of breads made with 100% whole wheat flour.

Super Nutrition Tip

While most Canadians have no problem eating the recommended 5 to 12 servings of grain products each day, we often fall short when it comes to choosing the "whole" grain options. That's why "3 is key" makes such good sense. Translated, this means: choose a minimum of 3 whole grain products each and every day.

Super Nutrition Tip

For added nutrition and fibre, use whole grain flours instead of refined flours when making muffins, cookies or breads. Guideline: 150 mL (2/3 cup) of whole wheat flour = 250 mL (1 cup) all-purpose flour. Try substituting half the flour first and see if you notice the difference.

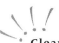

Clear the Confusion

There is no significant nutritional difference between unbleached and bleached flour. White flour is often bleached to give it a more consistent colour and to improve its baking qualities.

Perfect Spreads

The Sweet Stuff   Jams, jellies and honey are all fat-free. Although from a nutritional standpoint they contribute very little except calories, they make healthy foods taste better. What's more, when used as a replacement for high-fat hitters like margarine, butter and cream cheese, they can reduce your fat intake significantly.

The High-Fat Hitters   With 12 whopping grams of fat per tablespoon (15 mL), margarine and butter are the worst choices when it comes to spreading options. If, however, you limit your use to just 1 teaspoon (5 mL) of the stuff, you'll restrict the damage to 4 grams of fat. Better yet, use 1 teaspoon (5 mL) of fat-reduced margarine and cut your fat intake in half (about 2 grams of fat/tsp).

Cream Cheese Crusaders   At 5 grams of fat per tablespoon (15 mL), cream cheese contains less than half the fat in butter or margarine. There's only one problem: we tend to use it in such generous quantities. Best advice: use light cream cheese (3 grams of fat/tbsp) and spread it thin.

Pass the Peanut Butter   Peanut butter could never be called low in fat, as it contains 8 grams of fat per tablespoon (15 mL). However, it has something that most other spreads lack – some significant nutritional value, including protein, B vitamins, folic acid, phosphorus, magnesium, iron and even fibre (1 gram of fibre/tbsp). And unlike the artery-lining fat found in cream cheese and butter, peanut butter contains mostly monounsaturated fat (a hip-liner, but not an artery-liner). Therefore, if you lower your fat intake for the rest of the day, not only do you have room for peanut butter as a spread of choice, but you also get some great nutrition along with it.

The Bread and Spread Story

	Grams of fat
1 slice bread with butter or margarine (10 mL/2 tsp)	9.0
1 slice bread with peanut butter (15 mL/1 tbsp)	9.0
1 slice bread with cream cheese (15 mL/1 tbsp)	6.0
1 slice bread with jam (10 mL/2 tsp)	1.0
1 slice bread	1.0

Please note: Many people use 2 to 3 tablespoons (30–45 mL) of peanut butter or cream cheese per serving, as compared to the 1 tablespoon serving (15 mL) listed here.

News Flash: Bigger Bagels   Bagels are growing not only in popularity, but also in size. Unfortunately, as their size increases, many of us enter a "low-fat delusional state." We assume that since bagels are low in fat, even jumbo-size bagels can be eaten with reckless abandon. And yet, while a regular bagel contains about 200 calories, a jumbo bagel may contain in excess of 500 calories (not to mention the fact that the bigger the bagel, the more topping you spread on it).

Bottom line: too much food from any source can cause your waistline to expand.

4. Cereal and Milk: A Powerful Combination (Now this is exciting!)

You take the goodness of low-fat milk (the riboflavin, the calcium, the vitamin D) and the goodness of cereal (the iron, the fibre and all those spectacular B vitamins) and mix the two together and what have you got? Super nutrition in a bowl. Cereal and milk make a powerful combination when it comes to nutrition. What's more, if you choose wisely on the cereal front, you can increase your fibre intake significantly. Some bran cereals, for example, contain up to 10 grams of fibre in a mere $1/2$ cup serving (we're talking dynamite in a box). Which means that if you make high-fibre cereals a regular part of your day, reaching your daily 25-to-35-gram fibre quota becomes easy.

Super Nutrition Tip
Have cereal for breakfast. Studies show that cereal has fewer calories than other meals, like lunch or dinner, but still provides a lot of nutrition. Cereal can supply from 10 to 30% of your daily requirements for several key nutrients like vitamin B6, iron, calcium, magnesium, vitamin A, copper and zinc. All great reasons to be a lover of cereal!

Super Nutrition Tip
For extra nutrition and fibre, add some fruit to your cereal. While bananas are the most popular choice, dried fruits, like raisins or apricots, are also easy options. Berries in season (and on sale) are my personal favourite.

The Top Ten Cereal List
These brand name cereals are ranked in order of their fibre content.

		Grams of fibre
1.	Kellogg's Bran Buds with Psyllium	11.2
2.	Kellogg's All Bran/Post 100% Bran	10.1
3.	Post Fruit and Fibre	5.1–6.2
4.	Quaker Corn Bran	5.0
5.	Kellogg's/Post Raisin Bran	4.6–5.6
6.	Kellogg's/Post Bran Flakes	4.4–5.1
7.	Post Balance Multibran	4.2–5.0
8.	Weetabix	4.0
9.	Quaker Oat Bran Cereal	3.4
10.	Kellogg's Common Sense	3.1–4.1

Runners-Up List
containing at least 2 g of fibre per serving

	Grams of fibre
Kellogg's Muslix	2.4–3.9
Kellogg's Mini-Wheats	2.9
Quaker Life	2.8
Post Shreddies	2.7
Quaker Oat Squares	2.4
Instant Quaker Oatmeal	2.3–2.9
General Mills Cheerios	2.2
General Mills Oatmeal Crisp	2.1–3.0

Please note:
1. A range of fibre values is given for cereals with different flavours/varieties.
2. The fibre content is based on a 30-gram serving size (a small bowl).
3. Cereals that are high in fibre but not enriched with added vitamins and minerals (like Nabisco Shredded Wheat or Regular Oatmeal) have not been included on the list as they contain significantly less iron and fewer B vitamins (including folic acid) than their enriched counterparts. Both iron and folic acid are particularly important and often lacking in the diets of women.

Reduce the Fat

Granola sounds healthy, but the added nuts and oils make it much higher in fat than most other cereals. Even the new, lower-fat versions can be deceiving when you consider that the serving size, as represented on the side of the box, barely covers the bottom of a bowl. If you eat a decent-size bowl for breakfast, the fat grams consumed can easily exceed the 10-gram mark.

Taste Tip

If you don't like the taste of high-fibre cereals, mix them half and half with a cereal you do like. A Cheerios/All Bran combo is my favourite.

Super Nutrition Tip

Juice and cereal are a winning combination at the breakfast table. The vitamin C in the juice enhances the body's absorption of iron from the cereal.

"No man is lonely eating spaghetti; it requires so much attention."
Christopher Morley

5. Froot Loops Get a Passing Grade…Almost

Many people think sweetened cereals like Froot Loops or Frosted Flakes should be avoided at all costs. However, these cereals, when combined with milk, still offer a whopping dose of nutrition. Yes, they contain sugar, but except for its role in tooth decay and the extra calories it adds, sugar is not considered harmful to health. The biggest drawback to many of these sugary concoctions is their lack of fibre. But there are sweetened cereals out there that are also a good source of fibre. Golden Honey Shreddies, Multi-Grain Cheerios and Quaker Instant Oatmeal all contain at least 2 grams of fibre per serving. Better yet is Quaker Corn Bran with a hefty 5 grams of fibre per cup.

6. Pick the Right Pasta, Pick the Right Sauce

The right pasta, without question, is whole wheat pasta. And for the sauce, tomato sauce loaded with lots of veggies is about as good as it gets. Even the fattiest tomato sauces rarely go over 6 grams of fat in a

$^1/_2$ cup serving, whereas a typical cheese, Alfredo or pesto sauce can register well above the 30-gram mark per serving. Try to resist these higher-fat sauces most of the time. Better yet, try some of the reduced-fat versions found in this book (pages 191, 197, 199) and other healthy-eating cookbooks. Fatty meats like sausages or ground beef can also make a significant dent on the fat front when added to sauces. Ground beef is more acceptable if it is first browned and drained of all fat.

Read the Label
Not all pasta and noodles are enriched. Always look for iron, thiamin, niacin and riboflavin on the ingredient label when buying these products – particularly fresh pastas and Asian noodles.

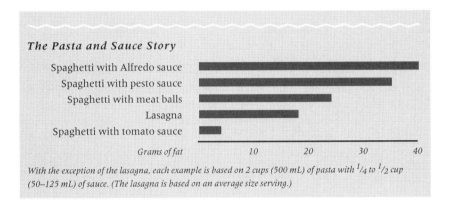

The Pasta and Sauce Story

	Grams of fat
Spaghetti with Alfredo sauce	
Spaghetti with pesto sauce	
Spaghetti with meat balls	
Lasagna	
Spaghetti with tomato sauce	

Grams of fat 10 20 30 40

With the exception of the lasagna, each example is based on 2 cups (500 mL) of pasta with $^1/_4$ to $^1/_2$ cup (50–125 mL) of sauce. (The lasagna is based on an average size serving.)

News Flash: No Veggies Don't expect much in the way of vegetables in premade tomato sauces. When the Centre for Science in the Public Interest picked apart a 28-ounce jar of Ragu Today's Recipe Garden Harvest, they found $^1/_6$ of a mushroom, $^1/_5$ of a carrot, $^1/_{17}$ of a green pepper, $^1/_{11}$ of an onion, $^1/_{16}$ of a celery stalk, $^1/_7$ of a zucchini, and 2 tablespoons of unidentifiable vegetable sludge. A vegetable garden in a bottle it's definitely not.

Reduce the Fat
Stay away from ramen noodles. When packaged in instant soup mixes, for example, they are precooked then dried by deep-frying in a highly saturated, artery-lining fat.

7. The World of Rice

From a nutritional point of view, short grain, medium grain and long grain rice are very similar. The main difference is their size. Most long grain white rice (the kind we eat the most of) is parboiled. Also known as converted rice, it is higher in nutritional value than regular white rice, as fewer nutrients are lost during processing. Better still is brown rice, which is whole grain.

Keep It Fresh
Brown rice comes in small boxes because the oil in the bran portion can go rancid if it sits around a long time before it is eaten. Store brown rice in the fridge if you plan to have it on hand longer than 6 months.

Reduce the Salt

Prepackaged rice and seasoning mixtures are taking up more and more shelf space at your local supermarket. They're fast, easy, and tasty. They are also high in salt and often higher in fat than regular rice (most contain about 4 to 6 grams of fat per ½ cup serving). To reduce the salt and fat content of these convenience products, use only half the seasoning-mix provided in the packet.

8. Pancakes, Waffles or French Toast?

Pancakes, waffles and French toast are all typically made with flour, eggs, oil and milk. It's the quantities of these ingredients, however, that influence the fat content of the final outcome. Generally speaking, pancakes are a low-fat choice, while waffles and French toast (particularly in a restaurant setting) can ring in at anywhere from 10 to more than 20 grams of fat in a typical serving. Some of the store-bought waffles, like Kelloggs Nutri-Grain Waffles, are lower in fat. The butter and syrup that go on top of any of these products can add to their fat and calorie content. I suggest you go easy on the butter or margarine ("bareback" pancakes – no butter or margarine – are always an option) and consider using one of the "light" syrups. All syrups are fat-free. However, light syrups contain about half the calories of regular syrups. Another suggestion: try plain or flavoured yogurt and fruit with pancakes.

> **News Flash: Tortillas** Tortillas are now sizzling hot in terms of popularity. Tortillas (and I don't mean tortilla chips, which are deep-fried) are low in fat and provide a great vehicle for making quick, nutritious meals. For example, fajitas, which are simply tortillas filled with stir-fried veggies and beans or lean meat, are healthy, quick and fun. Just be sure to go easy on the sour cream and guacamole.

The Muffin, Doughnut and Croissant Story

Based on typical serving size

	Grams of fat
Commercially bought muffin	18.0
Danish	18.0
Croissant	18.0
Doughnut	10.0
Homemade muffin	6.0

9. Muffins, Doughnuts, Croissants and All That Good Stuff

While grains are low in fat, some products made with grains – like muffins, doughnuts and croissants – are anything but. These delicious delights contain anywhere from 10 to 30 grams of fat per serving. While muffins can offer more fibre and nutrition than the others, most commercially made muffins are high in both fat and calories. Your best bet is a good old homemade muffin. Homemade muffins tend to be lower in fat, smaller in size and, depending on the recipe, often higher in fibre. What's more, homemade muffins freeze well. Make a big batch on the weekend and thaw them as you need them.

10. The Other Grains

For variety, why not step outside the regular arena of bread, rice and pasta? There is a multitude of other nutritious whole grains and grain products just waiting to add some exciting new tastes and textures to your next meal. Here are some of the possibilities: amaranth, barley, bulgur, buckwheat, couscous, millet and quinoa. Cooked bulgur and couscous are great in salads. Barley and amaranth add body to soups. Buckwheat and millet are a wonderful accompaniment to meats and vegetables. And quinoa is the perfect bed for sauces and other flavourful food mixtures. Most of these "other" grains get high marks on the nutritional front, with quinoa leading the pack.

Time Tip

If you love homemade muffins, but haven't the time to make them, try one of the low-fat muffin mixes. In most cases all you add is water (or milk for added nutrition), give a quick stir, and pop them in the oven. I usually add frozen blueberries or cut-up, canned fruit (like peaches, mmm) for extra taste and nutrition.

In a Nutshell...

Whole grains are important for the carbohydrates, B vitamins, iron, vitamin E and trace minerals they provide. The fibre found in whole grains is important for heart health, cancer prevention and weight management. Grains are naturally low in fat as long as they are not served with a high-fat spread or sauce. Eat 5 to 12 servings each day.

Four

Where's the Beef? (or Chicken or Pork?)

Three Things to Consider When It Comes to Eating Meat

1. Lean Meat Can Fit into a Healthy Diet

With all the bad press surrounding meat and health over the past few decades, are you wondering whether you should eat meat at all? An important question to answer is the following: Do people in those countries with the lowest rates of disease – from the Mediterranean to the Far East – eat meat? Yes! However, they don't eat meat in large quantities. Meat is not the main focus of the meal. And meatless meals, such as beans or fish, are also very common. This is consistent with studies that show meat can fit perfectly well into a healthy, well-balanced diet.

> **News Flash: Lean Meat**   Siberian reindeer herders eat two and a half times as much meat as the average North American, and yet they have much lower rates of heart disease. Why? Because they lead an active lifestyle and eat primarily reindeer meat, which is very, very lean.

Cancer Prevention
When fatty meat is barbecued over high heat, fat drips onto the heating element (coals, wood, gas flames, electric coils), forming potentially cancer-causing chemicals that are deposited on the meat by the rising smoke. Best advice: raise the grill as far from the coals as possible; don't barbecue every day; pick low-fat meats; trim all visible fat before cooking.

Serving Size Checklist
Canada's Food Guide to Healthy Eating recommends 2 to 3 servings of meat or meat alternatives (like beans, nuts or seeds) every day. One serving of meat is equal to 50 to 100 grams (2.0 oz–3.5 oz) of meat or poultry.

2. Meat Contains Artery-lining Saturated Fat

One of the keys to making meat fit into a healthy diet is to make sure it's lean. Certain cuts of meat, such as those used to make regular ground beef and many processed meats (sausages, bacon, wieners and certain luncheon meats) contain a significant amount of artery-lining saturated fat. If you eat too much of these products, your risk of both heart disease and certain cancers, like cancer of the colon and prostate, may be increased.

> **News Flash: Leaner Meat**   Beef and pork are up to 50% leaner today than they were 15 years ago.

3. Here Come Iron, Niacin, Vitamin B12, Protein and Zinc

If your diet is lacking in meat, which is more likely with women than men, you may not be getting enough vitamin B12, niacin or zinc, all of which are required for good health. Meat is an exceptional source of protein, a nutrient that is essential for building and maintaining our body tissues. Meat is also our most important source of heme iron (heme iron is the form of iron most readily absorbed by the body), another key nutrient that many women fail to get enough of.

Bottom line: meat has an important role to play in meeting our nutrient needs.

Six Super Tips on How to Be a Lean Meat Eater

1. Minimize Your Portion Size

It used to be that people ate meat and potatoes. Now it's time to eat potatoes and meat. In other words, it's time to make nutritious whole grains, fruits and vegetables the main event at every meal, while meat takes on a supporting role. One of the best ways to do this, other than loading up on the other foods, is to limit your serving of meat to the size of a deck of cards. To show you what a difference this makes, let's take a look at sirloin steak. If you eat a 100-gram (3.5-oz), deck-of-cards-size sirloin steak, you'll consume about 6.7 grams of fat. On the other hand, if you eat a 340-gram (12-oz) sirloin steak, like the kind found in most steak houses, you'll consume over 22 grams of fat. How much fat would you rather eat?

2. Trim The Fat...All of It

If you see any fat surrounding the edges of a steak or roast, cut it off. In doing so, you will significantly reduce your fat intake. As an example, a 100-gram (3.5-oz) serving of standing rib roast with the fat rings in at a whopping 20 grams of fat. The same amount of rib roast with the fat removed drops down to less than 11 grams.

3. Loin and Round Are Words to Watch For

Generally speaking, if you choose a loin or round cut of beef or pork, you will get a relatively low-fat cut of meat. Sirloin, sirloin tip, and tenderloin are all good examples of lower-fat loin cuts. Inside round, eye of round, and outside round are good examples of lower-fat round cuts. Because loin cuts are more tender, they can be cooked by broiling, grilling, or roasting on a rack. Round cuts are less tender and should either be marinated to tenderize prior to cooking or cooked using moist-heat methods such as braising or stewing. Beef short ribs and pork spareribs are among the fattiest cuts of meat.

Reduce the Fat
Instead of gravy or heavy sauces, serve your meat *au jus* (with just the juice from the meat), after skimming off all the fat. A quick way to remove the fat is to drop an ice cube into the cooled liquid. The fat will harden around the ice cube and can be easily removed.

Reduce the Fat
When broiling or roasting meat, always place the meat on a rack to allow the fat to drip away.

Read the Label
Canadian beef is rated from A to AAA as its marbling increases. "Marbling" refers to the fine white streaks of fat running throughout the lean portion of the meat. This marbling increases the tenderness, taste and juiciness of the meat, but it doesn't significantly influence the meat's overall fat content (the difference between 100 grams of triple-A beef and 100 grams of grade A beef is usually less than 1 gram of fat). You can therefore enjoy the superior eating quality of triple-A beef without worrying about the fat.

Taste Tip

You can tenderize a tough cut of meat with a kiwi. An enzyme in the fruit does the trick. Just cut the kiwi in half and rub it over beef, poultry or pork about 30 minutes before cooking. Or puree the fruit and use it as a marinade. Papayas contain a similar tenderizing enzyme.

Taste Tip

To tenderize lower-fat cuts of meat, marinate them in wine, lemon juice or tomato juice prior to cooking.

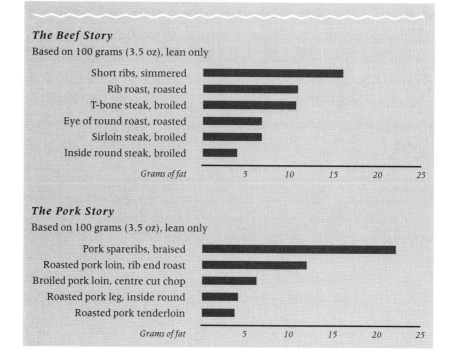

The Beef Story
Based on 100 grams (3.5 oz), lean only

Short ribs, simmered
Rib roast, roasted
T-bone steak, broiled
Eye of round roast, roasted
Sirloin steak, broiled
Inside round steak, broiled

Grams of fat　　5　　10　　15　　20　　25

The Pork Story
Based on 100 grams (3.5 oz), lean only

Pork spareribs, braised
Roasted pork loin, rib end roast
Broiled pork loin, centre cut chop
Roasted pork leg, inside round
Roasted pork tenderloin

Grams of fat　　5　　10　　15　　20　　25

Reduce the Salt

The sodium content of fresh meat is low. For example, freshly sliced turkey breast, chicken breast or roast beef are all low in salt. However, cured meats, such as ham, and most processed or prepackaged meats are very high in salt.

4. Lighten Up on Processed Meats

Depending on how much you eat, processed meats like bacon, sausages, hot dogs and certain luncheon meats can add a significant amount of artery-lining fat to your diet. Here are some suggestions to lighten up your choices:

Instead of...	Have...
Bacon/sausage	Ham
Hot dogs	Reduced fat hot dogs or veggie dogs
Bologna, salami, liverwurst	Lean ham, roast beef, turkey, chicken

Many companies now offer a low-fat line of luncheon meats. Schneiders Lifestyle luncheon meats is one widely available example.

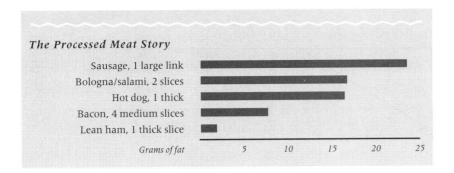

The Processed Meat Story

	Grams of fat
Sausage, 1 large link	
Bologna/salami, 2 slices	
Hot dog, 1 thick	
Bacon, 4 medium slices	
Lean ham, 1 thick slice	

5. The Ground Beef Dilemma

Let's start with the bad news. Contrary to popular belief, no ground beef, not even "extra lean" ground beef, is low in fat. What's more, ground beef (especially "regular" ground beef) can contribute a significant amount of artery-lining fat to your diet. Now for the good news. You can reduce the fat in ground beef added to foods like chili, spaghetti sauce and shepherd's pie by as much as half by browning the meat in a skillet and draining off all the fat. Rinsing the cooked meat in a strainer or colander with hot, not boiling, water will reduce the fat even further. When cooking hamburger patties, barbecue or broil on a rack rather than fry so that some of the fat drains away during cooking. Foods like meatloaf that lose little fat during the cooking process should always be made with "extra lean" ground beef and consumed in moderation.

Read the Label
Don't assume that a box of hamburger patties is low in fat just because the label reads "contains less than 10% fat." Meat is labelled based on the percentage of fat by weight, not the percentage of calories coming from fat.

Cooking Tip
When cooking ground beef, don't assume it's done simply because it looks brown. Some meat turns brown long before it is cooked sufficiently to kill dangerous bacteria such as E. coli. The colour of the meat's juices, not the meat itself, is a better indicator of doneness. The juices should change from red to nearly yellow.

The Ground Beef Story
Based on 100 grams (3.5 oz) meat

	100 g raw Grams of fat	100 g raw/broiled to well done Grams of fat
Regular ground beef	30	11.7
Medium ground beef	23	11.0
Lean ground beef	17	8.6
Extra lean ground beef	10	7.0

Please note:
1. One hundred grams of meat is about the size of 1 hamburger patty.
2. Each of the examples for raw meat is based on the maximum amount of fat allowed under current labelling regulations.
3. Depending on the cooking process used, the fat content of ground beef can be reduced by as much as a half.

Read the Label
Ground pork, chicken and turkey do not have to be labelled "lean," "medium" or "regular." If they are labelled, they must follow the same guidelines as ground beef (regular, no more than 30% fat by weight; medium, no more than 23%; lean, no more than 17%; and extra lean, no more than 10%).

Clear the Confusion
Don't assume that ground chicken or turkey is lower in fat than ground beef. Most ground chicken is made from thigh meat, which contains over three times as much fat as breast meat. What's more, the fat-laden skin of the chicken may also be ground up in the mix.

Reduce the Fat
While it's important to remove the skin from poultry, it makes little difference whether you do so before or after cooking. When roasting chicken, for example, leaving the skin on during cooking can help to retain the flavour, moisture and tenderness of the meat.

6. Breast Is Best/Trim the Skin

When it comes to poultry, here are two recommendations for low-fat living. Recommendation 1: Breast is best. Not only is white meat always lower in fat than dark meat, no other meat compares to chicken and turkey breast in terms of leanness. At the same time, if you really enjoy the taste of dark meat, it's my second recommendation that's most important. Recommendation 2: Trim the skin. I know, you've heard it before: always remove the skin from chicken. The reason? About two-thirds of the fat in poultry is in the skin! As an example, 100 grams of cooked chicken thigh without the skin contains 6.9 grams of fat as compared to 18.0 grams with the skin.

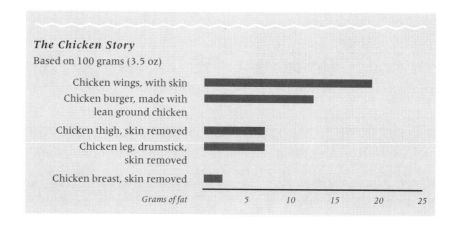

The Chicken Story
Based on 100 grams (3.5 oz)

	Grams of fat
Chicken wings, with skin	
Chicken burger, made with lean ground chicken	
Chicken thigh, skin removed	
Chicken leg, drumstick, skin removed	
Chicken breast, skin removed	

Grams of fat   5   10   15   20   25

A Word about Food Safety

Are There Chemicals in Our Food Supply?

Some medications, such as antibiotics, are approved for use in farm animals to prevent disease, treat sickness and improve growth. Withdrawal times and dosage levels, which have wide safety margins built into them, are established to make sure no detectable residues remain in the meat, eggs and dairy products we eat. Based on recent food inspection reports, 99.7 to 100% of the Canadian meat, milk and eggs tested for agricultural chemicals comply with Health Canada's strict laws.

> **News Flash: Mad Cow Disease**   On March 19, 1996, the health minister of the United Kingdom announced that BSE (bovine spogi-form encephalopathy) in cattle, also known as mad cow disease, may be linked to cases of a very rare human brain disorder called Creutzfeldt-Jakob disease. Both Canada and the United States have been declared BSE-free countries and regulations have been put in place to prevent mad cow disease from happening here.

Taste Tip
No butter, no oil, no herbs, just 2 lemons. Next time you are roasting a whole chicken, puncture 2 lemons in at least 20 places and place them in the cavity of the bird. Seal the opening with toothpicks and roast until done. Delicious!

Will Eating Meat Increase Our Resistance to Antibiotics?

Will eating meat from animals previously exposed to antibiotics increase our own resistance to antibiotics? First, while it is true that human resistance to antibiotics is increasing (in other words, antibiotics are becoming less effective), research to date indicates that eating meat plays little if any role in this development. Second, if resistant strains of bacteria do exist in the meat, proper cooking kills all harmful bacteria, resistant or not. To make sure that all bacteria are destroyed in the meat you eat, follow these guidelines:

1. Roasts and steaks can still be enjoyed rare (internal temperature 140°F/60°C) since any bacteria present are on the surface of the meat and killed quite readily.
2. Ground meat should be cooked to the well-done stage (internal temperature 170°F/75°C) as bacteria can be present throughout.

Taste Tip
The next time you bake chicken breasts in the oven, for a taste treat coat them first with one of the following low-fat ingredients: plain Dijon mustard, a honey-mustard mixture, a curry sauce, a mixture of Cajun spices or a prepared Hoisin sauce. Another option is to baste them with pureed fresh fruit (peaches, plums, cherries).

Clear the Confusion
Contrary to popular belief, chicken wings are not white meat. In fact, chicken wings are one of the highest-fat poultry choices – especially when you eat them skin and all.

In a Nutshell...

Beef, chicken and pork are important for the protein, iron, niacin, vitamin B12 and zinc these meats provide. Choose lean cuts of meats, trim the fat, watch your intake of processed meats (sausages, bacon, wieners and certain luncheon meats) and remove the skin from poultry to reduce your intake of artery-lining saturated fat. Eat 2 to 3 servings of meat or meat alternatives each day.

Five

Be a Fish Eater

Two Best Reasons in the World to Be a Fish Eater

Number One Best Reason: Heart-Healthy Omega-3s

What two things do the Greenlandic Inuit and the Japanese have in common? First, they both have rock-bottom rates of heart disease. Second, they eat a lot of food from the sea. So what's the connection between seafood and a healthy heart? The answer is *omega-3s*. Omega-3s are a type of fatty acid unique to seafood, especially fatty fish. Research indicates that when you eat fish containing omega-3s you reduce the stickiness of your blood. As a result, your blood is less likely to clot. Many heart attacks and strokes occur when blood clots get stuck in an already narrowed artery. In a recent study involving more than 2,000 middle-aged men, those who consumed at least 2 servings of fish per week reduced their risk of a heart attack by 29%. Other studies have reported risk reductions of as much as 50%. And that's not all. The benefits of omega-3s go beyond heart disease. Preliminary

Super Nutrition Tip
Although all fish contain *some* heart-healthy omega-3s, generally speaking, the fattier the fish, the more omega-3s they contain (yes, this is one time it's better to eat more fat). Herring, mackerel, trout, sardines, salmon and anchovies are all considered higher-fat, omega-3-rich choices. Lean fish, such as cod, haddock and sole contain much lower levels of omega-3s.

Clear the Confusion
Although vegetable sources of omega-3s, such as canola oil and flaxseed oil, do exist, their structure is somewhat different from the omega-3s found in fish. Researchers have yet to determine whether the vegetable source omega-3s are as beneficial to health as the type found in fish.

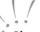

Clear the Confusion
Most frozen fish sticks and fast-food fish sandwiches are a poor source of omega-3s because of the type of fish used, and because some of the omega-3s are lost during processing.

Super Nutrition Tip
The omega-3 content of tuna varies considerably depending on the type you choose. Most of the fresh tuna on restaurant menus and at fish counters is yellowfin tuna, which is not high in omega-3s. A much better choice is bluefin tuna, which is served at some upscale restaurants. When choosing canned tuna, pick albacore tuna (usually labelled "white" tuna), which contains more omega-3s than other types.

research shows omega-3s may help alleviate inflammatory disorders such as rheumatoid arthritis and psoriasis. Omega-3s may also reduce cancer risk, particularly for breast, colon and prostate cancer. There is even some evidence that these heart-healthy fish oils can protect against asthma. Let's go fishing!

> **News Flash: Mothers-to-Be**   Pregnant and nursing women should regularly eat fish containing omega-3s, as these essential fats appear to play an important role in fetal and infant development.

Omega-3s in Pill Form

If omega-3s are so good for your health, why not pop them in a pill?

1. Many questions remain about the effectiveness and safety of omega-3 pills. No leading health or nutrition organization recommends them at this time.
2. Side effects from large doses include nausea, diarrhea, belching and a bad taste in the mouth.
3. Omega-3s in pill form provide a concentrated source of calories. Some recommended doses supply up to 200 calories per day. It's better to eat fish and get all the other wonderful nutrients – not to mention the pleasure – as well.

Conclusion: *Be a fish eater!*

Number Two Best Reason: Less Artery-lining Fat

Fish is an excellent choice for what it does contain – essential nutrients like protein, vitamin B12, niacin, magnesium, phosphorus, selenium and iron – but also for what it doesn't contain – a whole lot of artery-lining fat. That's right, all seafood is low in saturated fat. Most seafood contains less than 1 gram of artery-lining fat per serving (as long as it's not breaded, fried or mixed with huge quantities of mayo). Compare that to meats like beef, chicken or pork, which, depending on the cut, can contain up to five times as much saturated fat per serving.

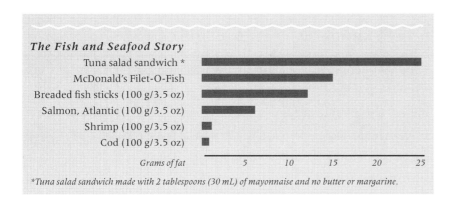

The Fish and Seafood Story

	Grams of fat
Tuna salad sandwich *	(approx. 25)
McDonald's Filet-O-Fish	(approx. 15)
Breaded fish sticks (100 g/3.5 oz)	(approx. 12)
Salmon, Atlantic (100 g/3.5 oz)	(approx. 7)
Shrimp (100 g/3.5 oz)	(approx. 1)
Cod (100 g/3.5 oz)	(approx. 1)

Grams of fat: 5 10 15 20 25

Tuna salad sandwich made with 2 tablespoons (30 mL) of mayonnaise and no butter or margarine.

Clear the Confusion
Contrary to grandma's advice, cod liver oil is not recommended. When taken in excess, it contains toxic levels of both vitamin A and vitamin D.

Six Fantastic Fish-eating Tips

1. Make It a Habit

Eat at least 2 servings of fish each week. Try to make sure one of these servings is rich in omega-3s. One serving equals 50 to 100 grams (2–3 oz) of fish, or one third to two thirds of a can.

2. Fish That Isn't "Fishy"

If you think fish tastes "too fishy," try some of the milder-tasting fish, like cod, haddock, halibut and orange roughy.

3. Learn How to Cook Fish

A lot of people don't eat fish because they don't know how to cook it. Try some of the fish recipes in this and other healthy-eating cookbooks. Experiment with one new fish recipe each month. The more you learn how to cook fish, the more you'll learn to love it.

Clear the Confusion
If you've been avoiding shellfish like shrimp because of its cholesterol content, listen up. First, more recent data indicates that all types of shellfish contain much less cholesterol than previously thought. Second, saturated fat, not cholesterol, is the main concern for heart health. Third, most people don't eat shellfish in large quantities or on a regular basis. Bottom line: enjoy your shellfish.

Cooking Tip
Don't overcook fish or it will get dry and tough. Most fish requires just 10 minutes of cooking time for each inch of thickness, making it an excellent choice for busy households. This rule applies whether you are baking, grilling, steaming, poaching or broiling your fish. Properly cooked fish will flake easily with a fork.

He was a bold man who first ate
an oyster.

Reduce the Fat

Rather than breaded and deep-fried
shrimp (fat gram city), may I suggest
shrimp simmered with lemon juice,
herbs and spices? Marinated shrimp
grilled on the barbecue or under the
broiler is another low-fat, tasty alternative. Last but not least, shrimp
cocktail gets two thumbs up, as the
cocktail sauce is low in fat and ever
so tasty.

Reduce the Fat

Make lower-fat tartar sauce by mixing
1 teaspoon (5 mL) of fat-reduced
mayonnaise with 1 tablespoon (15
mL) of relish.

4. Two Thumbs Up for Frozen Fish

A study at Pennsylvania State University compared the taste of fresh
fish to frozen fish. An expert panel of fish tasters ranked frozen cod
higher than fresh cod fillets purchased at local supermarkets. These
results are not surprising when you consider that frozen fish is often
frozen within four hours of being caught, whereas fresh fish sold in
supermarkets may be 10 days old by the time it's purchased. Frozen
fish is usually a lot cheaper too!

5. Please...Not the Breaded Kind

More than two thirds of the frozen fish consumed in Canada is sold in
breaded or battered formats. The problem is not the breading, but the
fact that the fish is deep-fried. Even the breaded fish fillets you bake at
home in the oven are deep-fried prior to packaging. As a result, a typical serving of breaded or battered fish is loaded with fat. Instead, try
High Liner's Healthy Bake, which is breaded fish that's baked, not
fried.

6. Watch the Mayo

Canadians eat more tuna than any other type of fish, and most of it is
canned. The problem with this is that we tend to eat it mostly in sandwiches mixed with lots of high-fat mayonnaise. In a recent sandwich
analysis, a typical mayo-heaped tuna salad sandwich rang in at a
whopping 56 grams of fat! Suggestion: whether at home or on the
town, have your sandwich with small quantities of reduced-fat mayo.

Are Fish and Seafood Safe to Eat?

Let's start with the good news. Many of the popular types of fish and seafood, like canned tuna, shrimp, cod, breaded fish fillets, fish sticks, flounder, haddock, catfish, and salmon (canned or fresh) are among the safest.

Polluted Water = Polluted Fish

Now the bad news: fish caught in polluted waters may contain accumulated chemical residues, such as mercury and lead. Inland rivers and lakes, including the Great Lakes, tend to be more severely polluted than the ocean, though some ocean shorelines are contaminated too. Generally speaking, freshwater fish like lake trout, bass, perch, pike and carp are more likely to be contaminated than ocean fish caught far offshore. This does not mean you have to avoid freshwater fish altogether. However, you should know where the fish came from. Much of the lake trout sold in supermarkets is perfectly safe since it comes from fish farms – commercially operated freshwater ponds, which are free of pollution. For more detailed information on whether fish caught from a particular area is safe, contact the Government of Canada, Fisheries and Oceans. Pregnant and nursing women should be particularly careful about avoiding contaminated fish.

Raw Seafood Is Risky

Eating raw seafood like sushi is a bit like playing Russian roulette. There's always a chance it may make you sick. Even the freshest fish may contain bacteria, parasites and other potentially harmful organisms. While it's true that well-trained sushi chefs know how to purchase and handle fish so as to minimize the risk of illness and parasitic infection, there is still no guarantee of safety. Raw shellfish such as

Reduce the Salt
Imitation crab meat, also called surimi, is made from white-fleshed fish like Alaskan Pollock. It is low in fat, but very high in salt.

Reduce the Fat
Always buy water-packed tuna. Tuna packed in oil contains up to five times as much fat.

Keep it Fresh
Smell is a good indicator of freshness when it comes to fish. Generally speaking, if it has a "fishy" odour, don't buy it. And cook fresh fish within 24 hours of purchase.

clams, oysters and mussels are particularly dangerous as they live by filtering 15 to 20 gallons of water a day. They can become a concentrated storehouse of bacteria and viruses.

Super Nutrition Tip
All shellfish, including clams, crab, oysters, lobster, mussels, shrimp and scallops, are low in fat and rich in protein, iron, copper and zinc.

In a Nutshell...

Be a fish eater. Fish and seafood are low in artery-lining saturated fat and are an important source of heart-healthy omega-3 fats. Watch out for the added fat found in fried and breaded fish and in tuna salad sandwiches. Fish caught in polluted waters and raw seafood may be unsafe.

Six

Have Eggs Instead?

Four Egg Facts You Should Know About

1. The Cholesterol Debate

Let's play the word association game. When I say "egg," what's the first word that pops into your mind? If you said "cholesterol," I wouldn't be surprised. Most of us have been programmed to think of eggs and cholesterol as one and the same. Here's what you need to know. First of all, eggs do contain cholesterol (about 200 milligrams per egg). Second, and more important, for most healthy individuals the amount of cholesterol in food has little or no effect on levels of blood cholesterol and the risk of heart disease. In a study at the University of Washington people ate 2 eggs a day for 12 weeks. At the end of the study, only those individuals who already had high levels of blood cholesterol when they entered the study showed significantly higher blood cholesterol levels. This is consistent with other research that shows some individuals (about 20–30% of the population) are more sensitive to the cholesterol in food than others. Dietitians usually sug-

Clear the Confusion
It's not the cholesterol in the food we eat that has the most effect on blood cholesterol levels. It's the artery-lining saturated fats found in foods like whole milk, full-fat cheeses, and fatty meats.

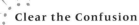

Clear the Confusion
Brown eggs offer no nutritional advantage over white eggs.

Reduce the Fat
To reduce the fat in fried or scrambled eggs, cook them in a good nonstick pan with a vegetable oil cooking spray rather than butter.

Super Nutrition Tip
Hens fed flaxseed are now producing omega-3-enriched eggs. Omega-3s, which are more commonly found in fish, appear to offer significant health benefits, including a reduction in heart disease risk. Researchers have yet to determine whether the vegetable source omegas are as beneficial to health as the type found in fish.

Super Nutrition Tip
Eggs are the ideal food for small appetites. In other words, they're great for kids.

gest that these high-risk individuals limit their cholesterol intake to 300 mg per day or less.

Bottom line: for most people – although the key emphasis should still be to eat more foods like fish, beans, whole grains, fruits and vegetables – eggs in moderation are perfectly acceptable.

2. One Egg Equals Five Grams of Fat

One egg contains 5 grams of fat, but only 1.5 grams of that are saturated. Once again, this means that eggs can be part of a healthy diet when eaten in moderation.

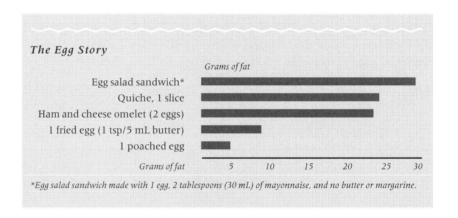

The Egg Story

Egg salad sandwich made with 1 egg, 2 tablespoons (30 mL) of mayonnaise, and no butter or margarine.

3. Nature's Multi-Vitamin in a Shell

Now for the beautiful side of the egg story. One egg contains a whole lot of nutrition. Eggs are what we dietitians call "nutrient dense." Within each and every egg you'll find high-quality protein, vitamin B12, vitamin E, vitamin A, vitamin D, riboflavin, folic acid, zinc, iron, phosphorus and more. In fact, you'll find just about every essential nutrient known to man, with the exception of vitamin C and a few trace minerals. That's pretty darned exceptional. It's also why the egg has been called "mother nature's all-purpose multi-vitamin."

4. Eggs for Dinner at Pennies a Plate

I rarely eat eggs for breakfast. Most mornings, I prefer the high fibre and nutrition of cereal. I'm more likely to eat eggs at dinnertime, especially on nights when I don't have time to cook a more elaborate meal. One egg, a couple of pieces of whole wheat toast, a glass of skim milk, and a piece of fruit makes for an extremely nutritious and inexpensive meal that can be prepared in minutes.

In an Eggshell... oops, I mean Nutshell...

Eggs contain a whole lot of nutrition in one little package. They are high in cholesterol, but contain only moderate amounts of saturated fat, which is the main offender when it comes to heart health. For most people, eggs in moderation can be part of a healthy diet.

Reduce the Fat
One fat-reducing technique that's recently come into vogue is eating only egg whites. While it is true that the yolk contains all the fat, it also contains most of the vitamins and minerals (egg whites contain mostly protein). It's therefore better to limit the number of eggs you eat rather than getting rid of the yolks altogether. Using egg whites instead of whole eggs to reduce the fat in baked goods is a more acceptable practice, since the baked goods are not usually the main source of nutrition for the meal.

Serving Size Checklist
Canada's Food Guide to Healthy Eating recommends 2 to 3 servings of meat or meat alternatives (like eggs) each day. One serving is equal to 1 or 2 eggs.

Seven

More Beans, Please!

Top Six Reasons to Say "More Beans, Please!"

1. The Standard to Judge All Others

If you were going to design the nutritionally perfect food, beans could be used as a standard to judge all others. They are chock-full of vitamins and minerals, including B vitamins, folic acid, zinc, potassium, magnesium, calcium and iron. They are the best plant source of protein and an excellent source of carbohydrates (the most efficient and preferred source of fuel for our bodies). They are so nutritious, in fact, that if the only change you made to your diet starting today was to eat more beans, you'd be making a significant difference.

2. Beans Are Low in Fat

With the exception of soybeans, beans are low in fat. An average cup of most beans contains less than 1 gram of fat. That's incredible. Even

Clear the Confusion
When I talk about beans, I'm really referring to the "legume" family. What exactly is a legume? Legumes are edible seeds enclosed in pods. The legume family includes dried peas (such as split peas, chickpeas and black-eyed peas), beans (such as lima, navy, kidney, pinto, black and soybeans), and lentils (such as red, brown and green lentils).

Super Nutrition Tip
Soybeans, pinto beans, chickpeas and lentils are among the most nutritious beans.

Reduce the Fat
Tofu, which is made from soybean curd, can vary considerably in its fat content. Generally speaking, firmer tofu is higher in fat, while softer, silkier tofu is lower in fat. Read the label and choose the lower-fat versions more often.

soybeans, which contain about 16 grams of fat per cup, contain primarily the heart-healthy unsaturated kind. In addition, most soy products, like soy milk and tofu, are available in lower-fat varieties.

3. A Fibre All-Star

When it comes to fibre, beans are second only to wheat bran in fibre content. Most beans contain about 9 grams of fibre per cup. Nine grams of fibre per cup is exceptional, especially when you consider that it's about one third of the recommended daily intake. In fact, when beans are a regular part of your diet, reaching your daily fibre quota is easy. Not only that, both types of fibre are found in beans. Insoluble fibre helps keep us regular and reduces the risk of colon cancer. Soluble fibre reduces the risk of heart disease by reducing the amount of cholesterol in our blood.

4. Potent Cancer Fighter

Although all beans are great, soybeans are one of the most nutritious foods known. They've been called the "king of the plant kingdom" and the "queen of the bean scene." And that's not all. In addition to their nutritional all-star status, soybeans are now gaining respect in the fight against cancer. In Japan, people who consume just 1 serving of soy a day are less likely to get cancer than those who don't. That's just 1 cup (250 mL) of soy milk or 4 oz (110 g) of tofu. Five different chemical classes of cancer fighters have been identified in soybeans including phytoestrogens, phytates, saponins, protease inhibitors and isoflavones. One of the most exciting compounds is a phytoestrogen called genistein, which shows great promise in blocking critical steps of the cancer process, particularly for hormone-related cancers like breast and prostate cancers. More beans, please!

5. Super Heart Protector

Beans, beans, they're good for your heart. Researchers from the University of Kentucky pooled data from 38 previous studies on soy. A daily intake of about 3 cups of soy milk or tofu was found to reduce blood cholesterol levels by an average of almost 10%. This translates into a 20% reduction in risk of heart disease. While 3 cups is more soy than most people are willing to eat, benefits were also seen at lower levels of intake, especially in those people who had the highest levels of blood cholesterol to begin with. Researchers believe that both the phytochemicals in beans and the soluble fibre play a role in protecting the heart.

Super Nutrition Tip
Roasted chickpeas make a great snack. Simply drain and rinse 1-540 mL (19 oz) can of chickpeas; place in bowl. Add 15 mL (1 tbsp) olive oil and 2 mL ($^1/_2$ tsp) each of salt and pepper; toss well to combine. Bake at 350 F (180 C), stirring occasionally, for about 1$^1/_2$ hours until golden and crisp. Each 50 mL ($^1/_4$ cup) serving contains 80 calories, 3 grams of fat, and 2 grams of fibre.

News Flash: Hot Flashes   The phytoestrogens found in soybeans and soy products may reduce some of the symptoms of menopause, such as hot flashes.

6. Nutritious Food Just Doesn't Get Any Cheaper

People who complain about the cost of healthful eating certainly couldn't be talking about beans. Beans are the nutritional bargain of a lifetime. In fact, replacing just a few meat meals each week with a few bean meals will result in a significant downward shift in your weekly shopping bill.

Super Nutrition Tip
Keep a few cans of beans – like chickpeas, kidney beans and black beans – in the cupboard at all times. That way, when you're looking for something to toss into a salad, soup or stew, you've got beans right at your fingertips. Frozen legumes are also widely available.

"Beans Give Me Gas" – Five Things You Can Do to Reduce the Hot Air

When I tell people about the nutritional superiority of beans, their first response is often, "What about the gas?" Unfortunate but true, one of the side effects of eating beans is flatulence caused by our inability to digest the raffinose sugars found in beans. Fortunately, we do have some control over the situation. Here are five great tips for reducing bean-induced hot air:

Serving Size Checklist
Due to their nutritional makeup, beans have been called "the meat that grows on vines." When you choose beans instead of meat, you get a great dose of nutrition without the saturated fat and with some extra fibre to boot. You should eat 2 to 3 servings of meat and alternatives (like beans) each day. One serving equals:
  125–250 mL (½–1 cup) of beans
  100 g (⅓ cup) of tofu
  250 mL (1 cup) soy milk/beverage
Remember, those countries with the lowest rates of both heart disease and cancer have a lot of "meatless" days.

1. Eat More Beans

That's right. Just by eating more beans our bodies adapt to a certain degree and less gas is the result.

2. Watch How You Cook Them

When cooking dried beans, never cook the beans in the water they've been soaked in as some of the raffinose sugars that cause the gas actually leach out into the water.

3. Drain and Rinse

Draining and rinsing canned beans will get rid of some of the sugars that cause gas.

4. Try Beano!

Beano, now widely available at supermarkets and drugstores, has been touted as a "social and scientific breakthrough." This product contains the enzyme that breaks down the hard-to-digest sugars in beans. Try it the next time you sit down to a plate of beans.

> **News Flash: Less Hot Air** In order to test the effectiveness of Beano, a product that reduces the gas caused by beans, volunteers were fed a bowl of chili with Beano and then a few weeks later chili without Beano. In each case, volunteers had to record their "flatulence events per hour" (what fun). At the end of the study the results were conclusive – chili plus Beano equals less hot air. Beans, anyone?

5. Eat Beans with Family and Friends

This is the easiest solution by far. Simply relax and enjoy your beans with those who know and love you best – eat beans with family and friends.

Seven Super Ways to "Up Your Bean Intake"

There are probably 101 different ways to eat beans, yet many of us are not quite sure just what to do with them or how to eat them. Not to worry. Here are seven super ways to increase your intake of this incredibly nutritious food.

1. Soup's Never Bean Better

Whether it's your grandma's favourite recipe or your own most recent concoction, a great way to up your bean intake is with soup. A wide selection of bean soups now line your supermarket shelves, including the convenient single-serving kind (just add water and eat). Choose the lower-sodium products when possible. Minestrone, split pea, or classic black bean soup are always great options when dining on the town.

2. Hummus Is for...Dipping

I love hummus. It's one of the easiest, tastiest, dippiest ways to eat beans. Hummus is made from mashed garbanzo beans – better known as chickpeas – and seasoned with garlic, lemon juice and olive oil. Use small wedges of whole wheat pita bread or vegetables like carrot sticks, green pepper strips and broccoli spears for dipping into hummus. Hummus also makes a great sandwich spread as an alternative to mayonnaise. Hummus contains about 3 grams of fat per tablespoon (15 mL) as opposed to the 11 grams found in a tablespoon of mayonnaise.

3. I Say Beans, You Say Chili

Make it spicy, make it mild, make it with kidney beans, make it with black beans, make it meatless, make it with meat. Just as there are 101 ways to eat beans, there are probably 101 ways to make chili. Chili is chock-full of beans and an all-time favourite for young and old. Chili is also great for making in big batches and freezing for later on when you don't have time to cook.

Reduce the Salt
Canned beans are a nutritious and time-saving alternative to cooking beans from scratch. Their only downside is their higher salt content. Most canned beans contain about 400 mg per $1/2$ cup. By draining the canning liquid and rinsing , however, you'll cut the salt by almost half.

Super Nutrition Tip
When it comes to beans, hummus is not your only dipping option. Other bean dips are equally tasty and widely available. Black bean dip is one of my favourites.

4. Baked Beans Are the Best

Did you know that July is National Baked Bean Month? Well, you don't have to wait until July to enjoy the taste and nutrition of baked beans. Make them from scratch (forget the lard, bacon and other fatty recipe additions, use lean ham instead) or buy canned baked beans. When buying canned baked beans, your healthiest choice is beans in a plain tomato sauce.

5. Sensational Bean Salads

Bean salad – if you haven't had beans in a salad lately, you're missing out one of the most wonderful opportunities to up your bean intake. Cold salads, hot salads, beans mixed with greens, beans mixed with pasta, beans mixed with rice – the combinations are truly endless. Try one today.

6. Terrific Tofu

Tofu, often called "the cheese of Asia," is probably the most versatile ingredient in the soybean family. Tofu's greatest asset is its bland flavour. It absorbs the flavours of the foods it's cooked with or marinated in. Tofu can be stir-fried, broiled, grilled, or sautéed. It can be added to soups, stews, casseroles, salads, and even baked goods. It can substitute for part of the cheese in pizza or lasagna recipes. Last but not least, tofu, especially the soft and silken variety, is great for blending into shakes, salad dressing, dips and spreads. Sneak it into pasta sauces, scrambled eggs, macaroni and cheese, chili and so on.

7. *Soy City*

Besides tofu, there are a multitude of soy-based products on the market, including miso (soybean paste), tempeh (fermented soybean), soy flours, soy milk, roasted soybeans and soy-meat substitutes like veggie hot dogs, veggie burgers and soy ground beef replacement. Make it a habit to try at least one new soy product or soy recipe each month.

Super Nutrition Tip
Get yourself a good bean cookbook, like Kay Spicer's *Full of Beans*, and start benefiting from the high calibre nutrition of beans today.

In a Nutshell...

Beans belong on the nutritional powerhouse list. They are low in fat, high in fibre, and packed with vitamins and minerals. Beans, particularly soybeans and soy products, contain important compounds that can reduce the risk of both heart disease and cancer.

Eight

Sometimes I Feel Like a Nut

Four Nutty Things about Nuts

1. Nut Nutrition

If you're nuts about nuts, you'll be glad to know that they contain many nutrients essential to good health. Ounce for ounce, they are among the best plant sources of protein. They are rich in fibre and provide plenty of folic acid and other B vitamins. In addition, nuts contain iron, selenium, copper, zinc, potassium and magnesium. In a nutshell, they are chock-full of nutrition.

Super Nutrition Tip
Many of the nutrients found in nuts (like vitamin E, folic acid, iron and zinc) are lacking in the diets of many Canadians.

2. Fat Gram Overload

Although high in nutrition, nuts are also loaded with fat. In fact, about 70 to 95% of the calories in most nuts and seeds comes from fat. Just a couple of handfuls contain almost 40 grams of fat. That's a lot of fat, especially when you consider that women should consume no more than 65 grams of fat in a day and men no more than 90 grams.

Reduce the Fat

"Chestnuts roasting on an open fire" (you're supposed to sing that part). Out there in the world of high-fat nuts, there actually exists one, and only one, low-fat nut – the chestnut. One serving of roasted chestnuts, about 1/2 a cup, contains a mere 1.6 grams of fat. Now that's something to sing about.

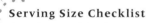

Serving Size Checklist

Canada's Food Guide to Healthy Eating recommends 2 to 3 servings of meat or meat alternatives (like nuts) each day. One serving equals:

30 mL (2 tbsp) nuts or seeds
30 mL (2 tbsp) peanut butter

3. It's Hip-Lining Fat

A half cup of most nuts contains more than 400 calories. In other words, too many nuts equals too big a waistline. Fortunately, the news is not all bad. With the exception of the coconut, nuts are not a concern when it comes to clogging your arteries. That's because most nuts contain primarily heart-healthy monounsaturated fats as opposed to the notorious artery-lining saturated kind. In fact, several studies suggest that regular nut eaters have a lower risk of heart disease.

4. The Best Way to Eat Them

I have two thoughts for fellow nut eaters. First, be good to your waistline and eat nuts in small quantities. Second, rather than eating nuts the way most people eat them – as a salty snack – eat them as a replacement for meat. The perfect example is a peanut butter sandwich. More possibilities: you can add nuts to casseroles, stir-fries, salads or rice. By replacing meat with nuts, you'll reduce your intake of artery-lining saturated fat. Just be sure to limit your serving of nuts to about 30 millilitres (2 tbsp).

Three Things Lovers of Peanut Butter Should Know

1. Peanut Butter May Not Be for Dieters, but Junk Food It's Not

Like nuts, peanut butter contains both a lot of nutrition and a lot of fat. That's why the same advice applies to both: Eaten in moderation, they can be part of a healthy diet.

2. "Light" Is not "Low-Fat"

Don't forget that "light" does not mean "low-fat." Light peanut butter contains about 12 grams of fat per serving (30 mL/2 tbsp), whereas regular contains 16 grams. In other words, peanut butter of any kind makes a substantial contribution on the fat front. The best advice no matter what the brand: spread it thin.

> **News Flash: Peanut Butter** Ninety-two per cent of children eat peanut butter at least twice a week.

Food Allergy Tip
Women with a family history of allergies may be wise to avoid peanuts during the last three months of pregnancy and while breastfeeding, to reduce their child's risk of developing an allergy to peanuts.

3. Natural versus Commercial Brands

Is it better to buy "natural" peanut butters or commercial brands? The answer isn't easy. It's true that artery-lining hydrogenated fat is added to commercial peanut butters in order to keep the oils naturally present from separating, but most of the fat is still the monounsaturated heart-healthy kind. It's also true that commercial brands generally contain added salt and sweeteners, but again, the amounts are not significant. In addition, all natural peanut butters must be refrigerated to maintain freshness and to help prevent the oils from separating.

In a Nutshell...

Nuts provide lots of nutrition, but are high in fat. The fats are, however, primarily the heart-healthy kind. Nuts, including peanut butter, can be part of a healthy diet when eaten in moderation.

Nine

Take a Ride on the Low-fat Milky Way

Four Totally Terrific Reasons to Be a Lover of Milk and Milk Products

1. A Whole Lot of Nutrition in a Small Amount of Food

Without question, milk and milk products deserve a place on the nutritional all-star list. Based on a review by the National Institute of Nutrition, if you don't regularly consume milk products, you are unlikely to get enough calcium, riboflavin, vitamin D, vitamin A and vitamin B12. Milk provides all these nutrients, along with protein, phosphorus, magnesium, potassium and zinc. That's why a glass of milk in the middle of a hectic day goes a long way toward helping you meet your daily nutritional needs.

2. Build Your Bones with Calcium

Your spouse gives you a hug. You step off a curb. You pick up a heavy bag of groceries. If you suffer from osteoporosis, any of these simple actions could cause your bones to break. Osteoporosis, which is char-

Super Nutrition Tip
Milk can be substituted for water in most recipes, including such foods as pancakes, muffins and most baked goods. Milk also gives a great nutritional boost to hot cereals, like oatmeal. Don't water down your food!

Clear the Confusion
Contrary to popular belief, skim milk is not watered down when it comes to nutrition. It contains just as much calcium and other important nutrients as other types of milk. The main difference is the fat content.

Taste Tip

Chocolate milk contains all the wonderful nutrients found in regular milk, with some wonderful taste to boot. Chocolate powder or syrup adds a few extra calories, but hardly any fat.

Mouth On Fire!

Do you like your food hot and spicy? If so, the next time your mouth is on fire, cool it off with a glass of milk. Milk contains a protein known as casein, which is particularly effective at washing away the substance in hot peppers that causes the burning sensation.

Reduce the Fat

Most people find if they take it slow they can easily switch to lower-fat milk. If you drink 2% milk, make the switch to 1% milk first and then, once adjusted, get ready to take the skim milk plunge.

acterized by fragile or brittle bones, affects mostly women (1 of 4 women will have an osteoporosis-related fracture in her lifetime), although men are not immune. Both children and adults can reduce their risk of this truly debilitating disease by consuming a diet rich in calcium. The best source of calcium is dairy products.

Bone Health and Kids

Many studies have reinforced the significance of calcium early in life, a time when bone tissue is still forming. One study involved 70 pairs of twins, aged 6 to 14. The twins were split into two groups. One group consumed significantly more calcium than the other. Not surprisingly, the high calcium group showed significant increases in the density of their bones.

> **News Flash: Better Bones** It pays to drink more milk. Studies suggest that a lifetime of sufficient calcium intake results in a reduced risk of fracture later in life of between 20 and 60%.

Bone Health and Adults

Calcium does little to build bones in individuals over the age of 30, but it does maintain the bone that is already there and prevent further losses from taking place. In a study from France, elderly women had 43% fewer fractures when they increased their calcium intake.

> **News Flash: Better Bones** New studies suggest that getting enough calcium in the middle years really does make a difference. Based on a review of 33 studies, women who took in an extra 1,000 milligrams of calcium a day hung on to 1% more bone every year than women who didn't.

3. Vitamin D: The Other Bone Builder

Although most people know calcium is important for bone health, they are unaware of the importance of vitamin D. And yet without adequate vitamin D, the calcium we consume is not as well absorbed.

Although our body makes vitamin D when sunlight strikes our skin, in Canada's northerly latitude we could sit naked on our roofs all winter long (I don't recommend this) and still not produce any. Even in summertime, thanks to the regular use of sunscreens, the production of vitamin D by the skin may be minimal (this is particularly so for the elderly and young children). That's why food sources of vitamin D are so important. Unfortunately, the only natural sources of vitamin D are liver, fish and eggs. Vitamin D is therefore added to all milk and margarine (making diseases like rickets a thing of the past). What many people don't realize, however, is that vitamin D is not added to milk products like yogurt, cheese or ice cream – only to fluid milk.

4. Yogurt: More Than Just Nutrition

Yogurt is fast establishing itself as a nutraceutical, a food with health benefits beyond its nutritional value. Live bacterial cultures, such as lactobacillus bifidus, lactobacillus acidophilus and lactobacillus casei, are added to yogurt during processing. These live cultures help us to maintain a healthy gastrointestinal tract. They appear to stimulate the immune system and also help to prevent and treat gastrointestinal problems, such as certain types of diarrhea. When buying yogurt, look for the phrase "live cultures" or "active cultures" on the ingredient label (in some yogurts the live cultures are killed during processing). The future will tell us more about the health-enhancing benefits that yogurt may provide.

Milk Products Are Great IF...

When it comes to the nutritional value of milk products, there is one important exception to the rule. Milk products are great if . . . they are low in fat. Ideally, you want to get all the goodness of milk – all those wonderful vitamins and minerals – without the artery-lining saturated fat that often comes along for the ride. Here are a few suggestions for enjoying milk products the low-fat way:

Clear the Confusion
What is fresh cheese? Although nearly all cheese is made from milk solids (curds), some cheeses are aged or ripened, while others are not. Fresh cheese is soft, unripened cheese. It is much milder in flavour and usually lower in fat than most ripened cheeses. Cottage, ricotta, and quark cheese are all examples of fresh cheese. Minigo and Petit Danone are examples of fresh cheese products for kids.

Super Nutrition Tip
Relatively new to the market are low-fat fresh cheese products, like Danone Passion and Yoplait Caresse, that come in flavours like strawberry, maple, raspberry and vanilla. Their mild taste and thick consistency make them an ideal healthy snack, a delicious dessert, a great topping for fruit salad, a wonderful spread for bagels or toast and a tasty topping for cold or hot cereal.

Reduce the Fat
A great replacement for cream in most recipes and in your coffee is evaporated milk.

Suggestion 1. Buy 1% (or Less) Milk

Milk labelling is based on the percentage of fat by weight. For example, 2% milk contains 2% fat by weight. (It is not labelled, as some people think, by the percentage of calories coming from fat. If this were the case, 2% milk would be referred to as 35% milk, as 35% of its calories come from fat.) Your best bet is to stick with either 1% milk or skim milk. And use milk in your coffee instead of fat-laden cream.

Suggestion 2. Cheese: Not Too Much and Lower Fat

It's time to take a serious look at our cheese-eating habits. Cheese is the number one source of artery-lining fat in the Canadian diet. This doesn't mean we have to avoid eating cheese altogether. It means we should eat cheese in smaller quantities and choose the fat-reduced varieties more often. Get in the habit of checking cheese labels for percentage of milk fat. Low-fat cheeses, such as skim milk cheese, contain 7% M.F. (milk fat). Most "light" cheeses contain about 15% M.F. Full-fat cheeses, on the other hand, contain 30 to 35% M.F. And remember, many low-fat cheeses have improved significantly in taste.

Suggestion 3. Buy Low-Fat Brands

Buy the reduced-fat brands of yogurt, sour cream, cottage cheese or ice cream whenever possible. With yogurt and cottage cheese, stick to brands that contain 2% or less M.F.

Dairy Type

Dairy Type	Percentage of Calories from Fat
Coffee cream	86
Homogenized milk	49
2% milk	35
1% milk	23
Skim milk	5

The Milk Story

Based on a 250 mL (1 cup) serving

	Grams of fat
Homogenized (whole) milk	8.6
2% milk	5.0
1% milk	2.7
Skim milk	5

Please note: Most of the fat in milk products is the artery-lining saturated kind.

Taste Tip

If you prefer milk with a richer, creamier taste, try one of the more recent additions to the milk scene, like Neilson's Trutaste or Beatrice Plus. These products get their creamy taste from added milk solids, which provide extra taste and nutrition, but not extra fat. For some people, these products make the switch from 2% milk to either 1% or skim just that much easier to take.

The Cheese and Yogurt Story

	Grams of fat
Cheddar cheese, 33% M.F. (50g/3x1x1 in)	17.0
Partly skimmed mozzarella cheese, 18% M.F. (50g/3x1x1 in)	9.0
Cream cheese, 30% M.F. (15 mL/1 tbsp)	5.0
Cottage cheese, 1% M.F. (250 mL/1 cup)	2.7
Yogurt, .4% M.F. (250 mL/1cup)	1.0

News Flash: CLA Fights Cancer Just when you thought nutrition couldn't get any more confusing, along comes CLA (conjugated linoleic acid). It ranks among the most potent cancer fighters ever identified. It is found mainly in the fat of milk and beef. Researchers are investigating ways of increasing its concentration in dairy products so that we can enjoy its possible cancer-fighting benefits without having to consume large quantities of milk fat and thereby increase our risk of heart disease.

Five Top Misconceptions about Milk Products

Myth 1. I Can Get All the Calcium I Need from Other Sources

Many people are under the impression that they can get all the calcium they need from foods like dark green leafy vegetables, nuts, seeds, and beans. They can – as long as they are willing to eat these foods by the truckload (slight exaggeration) and on a daily basis. What's more, it's important to recognize that the calcium in dairy products is absorbed better than the calcium from most other foods.

Amount of Food Required to Replace the Amount of Calcium in 1-8 oz or 250 mL Glass of Milk

250 mL (1 cup) of almonds OR
575 mL (2⅓ cups) of sesame seeds OR
625 mL (2½ cups) of broccoli OR
175 mL (¾ cup) of kale OR
50 mL (⅔ cup) of tofu (made with calcium) OR
7,875 mL (31½ cups) soy beverage OR
2,875 mL (11½ cups) of kidney beans

Please note: This list is based on the amount of calcium absorbed by the body.

Myth 2. Most People Don't Tolerate Milk

Some people have problems digesting lactose, the sugar in milk. These people have low levels of the enzyme lactase. This intolerance (the

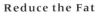

Reduce the Fat
Before you pile a heap of whipped cream on your pumpkin pie, consider this: 1 cup (250 mL) of whipped cream contains 44 whopping grams of fat.

Reduce the Fat
A light sprinkle of Parmesan cheese on your pasta contains only 2 grams of fat. Reduced-fat Parmesan cheese is also now widely available with a mere 1 gram of fat per tablespoon (15 mL).

Reduce the Fat
One tablespoon (15 mL) of butter contains 12 grams of fat. One tablespoon (15 mL) of sour cream contains 2.5 grams of fat. As long as you don't use sour cream by the bucketful, it's the better choice. Use a fat-reduced sour cream and you'll be even further ahead.

Super Nutrition Tip
Cow's milk should not be given to babies under 1 year of age. It contains too much of some nutrients and too little of others. While breast milk is definitely the ideal food, infant formulas, including those made from cow's milk, are the best alternative.

Clear the Confusion
Soy milk (the proper term is soy beverage), although a great food choice (see section on beans), is in no way a replacement for cow's milk. In fact, just the term "soy milk" is misleading. Soy milk is really not a milk at all. It is made from grinding soybeans with water. Cow's milk contains significantly higher levels of many nutrients, including vitamin A, riboflavin and vitamin B12. More important, soy milk is not a good source of calcium and contains no vitamin D whatsoever.

Clear the Confusion
If you or your child has a cold, there is absolutely no reason to avoid milk or dairy products. Contrary to popular belief, studies have found no connection between milk or other dairy products and mucus formation.

Cow's Milk Versus Goat's Milk
Although goat's milk is equal to cow's milk in terms of calcium, cow's milk is superior overall. Goat's milk is not always available in low-fat varieties, nor is it fortified with vitamin D. And goat's milk is significantly lower in both folic acid and vitamin B12. In addition (contrary to popular belief), for the small percentage of people allergic to cow's milk, two thirds will also be allergic to goat's milk.

proper term is maldigestion), however, is not as common as most people think. In addition, a recent study from Minnesota indicates that people who suffer from it have no problem drinking 1 cup of milk per day. In fact, it is only when milk is consumed in large quantities and at one sitting that it is cause for concern. In any case, if you suffer from lactose intolerance consider the following four tips:

Four Tips for Dealing with Lactose Intolerance

Tip 1. Drink milk with meals in small amounts, such as half-cup servings, spaced throughout the day.

Tip 2. Choose cheese and yogurt more often. Cheese, particularly hard cheeses like cheddar, contains almost no lactose. Yogurt contains an enzyme that digests much of the lactose present.

Tip 3. Lactose-reduced milks, like Lactaid, and tablets you add to your milk to break down the lactose can be used to boost your milk intake.

Tip 4. Increase your milk intake gradually. Most people can adapt to milk if they take it slow.

Myth 3. It's Unnatural to Drink Milk

Some people believe that drinking cow's milk is unnatural. But in much the same way as we harvest crops to survive, we take the milk of other animals for the unique and exceptional advantages it offers.

Myth 4. People from Other Parts of the World, Like Asia, Don't Drink Milk and Don't Get Osteoporosis

First, it is a myth that people in Asia do not suffer from osteoporosis. In fact, the incidence of hip fractures has increased dramatically in many Asian countries. Their low intake of calcium combined with a significant decrease in their day-to-day levels of physical activity (also a key risk factor for osteoporosis) are to blame. Second, many factors, including lifestyle, genetics and overall diet, influence both the risk of osteoporosis and the need for calcium. For example, a high salt intake, which is typical of the North American diet, can increase the need for calcium. Third, and most important, even when all diet and lifestyle factors are considered, adequate calcium intake is still an essential component of optimal bone health for all.

Myth 5. Milk Causes Everything from Ear Infections to Acne

You name it, milk has been blamed for it. Yet none of the popular "milk bashing" statements can be supported by scientific fact. In contrast, the recommendation that people of all ages should consume milk products is founded on sound principles of nutrition and comprehensive reviews of the most current research in the field.

How Much Milk Should I Drink?

Now that I've convinced you (at least, I hope I have) that milk and milk products are essential for good health, let's take a look at how much we should consume on a daily basis.

Preschoolers, 2–5 years	2–3 servings
Children, 4–9 years	2–3 servings
Youth, 10–16 years	3–4 servings
Adults	2–4 servings
Pregnant and breastfeeding women	3–4 servings

Please note:
1. Consume at least half of your dairy intake in the form of fluid milk to make sure your vitamin D requirements are met.
2. People with higher calorie needs should consume the higher number of recommended servings.
3. Most health experts recommend that postmenopausal women consume 4 servings per day. With age, decreasing estrogen levels increase the loss of bone tissue.

Clear the Confusion
What is filtered milk? Filtered milk, like Lactantia PurFiltre, goes through an additional step, called micro-filtration, beyond pasteurization. Filtered milk has a longer shelf life than regular milk – 30 days as opposed to 16 to 20 days. Some people also prefer the taste.

Serving Size Checklist
Each serving of milk products contains at least 275 mg of calcium.

The following amounts of food would be equal to 1 serving:
250 mL (1 cup) of milk
50g (3x1x1 in or 2 slices) of cheese
175g (¾ cup) yogurt
45 mL (3 tbsp) Parmesan cheese

The following amounts would be equal to ½ serving:
175 mL (¾ cup) ice cream
125 mL (½ cup) frozen yogurt
250 mL (1 cup) cottage cheese

Clear the Confusion
Despite its name, buttermilk contains no butter. In fact, most buttermilk is made from skim or 1% milk and is a low-fat, healthy choice. Buttermilk also adds great taste and texture to many low-fat recipes.

It's Easier Than You Think

Meeting your needs for calcium can be easier than you think. For example, start your day with a café au lait made with skim or 1% milk. Have milk on your cereal. Enjoy milk in your coffee or tea throughout the day. Have a slice of low-fat cheese in your sandwich at lunch. Have some yogurt as a snack in the afternoon. Have a glass of milk with your dinner. Sprinkle some Parmesan cheese on your pasta. Have a bowl of frozen yogurt for dessert. It's that easy!

Super Nutrition Tip

One cup of cottage cheese contains about half the calcium you'd find in a glass of milk or a container of yogurt. Cream cheese, which is mostly fat, contains almost no calcium at all.

Recommended Calcium Intakes

Age	Mg/Day
1–3	500
4–8	800
9–18	1300
19–50	1000
51+	1200

News Flash: Girls Swapping Milk For Diet Soft Drinks!

Around the age of 12, weight-conscious girls start swapping their milk for diet soft drinks. A new drink on the market, called Calais, is made with sparkling water and comes in such flavours as blackberry, raspberry and mandarin orange. These bottled waters have only 6 calories per serving, and more important, they contain 300 mg of calcium per 300 mL (10-oz) bottle. While these drinks are certainly a better choice than soft drinks, they still can't compare to the overall nutritional goodness of milk.

Should I Take a Supplement ?

If you do not consume the recommended number of servings of dairy products, you should consider a calcium supplement. If you don't consume at least half of your servings of milk products in the form of fluid milk, you should also consider a supplement for vitamin D (see section on supplements on p. 137 for more information).

Reduce the Salt

One of the main advantages of processed cheese spreads and slices is their convenience. However, from a nutritional standpoint, one of the main disadvantages of these products is their high salt content and somewhat lower nutritional content. The best advice is to use them in moderation and choose the lower-fat versions where possible. (If a little bit of Cheez Whiz Light melted in the microwave and poured over broccoli makes this wonderfully nutritious vegetable ten times as appealing to your kids, that's great.)

In a Nutshell...

Milk products are an important source of many nutrients, including riboflavin, vitamin A, vitamin B12, vitamin D and calcium. Both vitamin D and calcium are important throughout life to build and maintain healthy bones and to prevent osteoporosis. Choose lower-fat milk products to reduce your intake of artery-lining saturated fat. The many myths associated with milk drinking are not supported by scientific fact. Consume 2 to 4 servings each day.

Ten

To Be or Not to Be ...a Vegetarian

Five Things to Be Aware of When It Comes to "Vegging Out"

1. It Can Be Healthier

Vegetarians tend to have lower rates of obesity, heart disease, hypertension, diabetes and some cancers. That's because a good vegetarian diet is rich in health-enhancing foods like fruits, vegetables and whole grains, while also low in artery-lining saturated fat. Not all vegetarian diets, however, are the same. There are well-balanced, nutrient-rich vegetarian diets, and there are unbalanced, nutrient-poor vegetarian diets. For some teens, for example, "vegetarian" means bypassing the hamburger and just eating the fries, which is neither healthy nor balanced. In the end, meat or no meat, it's the quality of the overall diet that is most important.

Super Nutrition Tip
Healthy vegetarian eating means planning what you eat very carefully. The more foods you decide to cut out, the harder you have to work to meet your nutrient needs.

2. It Doesn't Have to Be All or Nothing

If you are considering the switch to a vegetarian diet, keep in mind that it doesn't have to be all or nothing. Some people omit all meat products from their diet, others continue to eat chicken or fish and still others eliminate eggs and dairy products as well as meat and fish. None of these is right or wrong. Whichever route you choose, your objective should be to eat a well-rounded, high-fibre, low-fat diet.

3. Don't Forget to Replace the Meat

When you remove the meat from a meal, it's important to replace it with foods that have a similar nutrient profile. It all comes down to three key words – beans, nuts and seeds.

4. Are You Getting Enough Vitamin B12, Vitamin D, Calcium, Iron and Zinc?

Generally speaking, the more restrictive a person's diet, the harder they have to work to get all their nutrients. All vegans, for example, should take a vitamin B12 supplement or eat foods fortified with vitamin B12, since this nutrient is found only in animal products. For those vegetarians who choose to avoid milk products, a supplement of vitamin D and calcium is often recommended. Both iron and zinc may also be less than adequate in a vegetarian diet. Although beans and whole grains are a good source of both nutrients, the vegetarian who eats some eggs, chicken or fish will find it easier to meet his or her requirements. Pregnant and breastfeeding women should be particularly careful to ensure all of their nutrient needs are met.

5. Children and Vegan Diets

Severe malnutrition, as well as deficiencies of iron, vitamin B12, calcium and vitamin D have been reported in infants and toddlers fed inappropriate vegetarian diets. Generally speaking, strict diets in which all animal products are omitted are not recommended for children. Children need lots of calories and nutrients for proper growth and development relative to their small size. To follow a "vegan" diet, kids have to eat a larger volume of food to meet their needs. Unfortunately, they often get full before their needs are met. A lacto-ovo-vegetarian diet, in which milk products and eggs are included, is more likely to meet the needs of growing children. Teenagers, who are increasingly turning to a vegetarian way of life, should be encouraged to visit a dietitian to learn the essentials of healthy eating, vegetarian style.

In a Nutshell...

A well-balanced vegetarian diet that is rich in whole grains, fruits and vegetables and low in artery-lining saturated fat is a healthful way to eat – as long as meat is replaced with foods that contain similar nutrients, such as beans, nuts and seeds. A supplement may be required for vitamin B12, calcium and vitamin D. Children should not be placed on a strict vegetarian diet.

Clear the Confusion

Contrary to popular belief, vegetarians can meet their protein needs by eating a variety of grains, nuts, seeds and beans throughout the course of a day. In the past, it was believed that certain food combinations, like corn and beans (complementary proteins), were required at the same meal.

Time Tip

When your teenage daughter is the only vegetarian in the family, how can you serve dinner without cooking 2 meals? Serve family entrees in which meat won't be missed, such as lasagna, quiche or pizza. Partly cook pasta sauces and stir-fries, and separate a portion for the non-meat-eater before adding meat. Double up when making vegetarian dishes, and freeze half to serve to your teen when meat is on the menu. Better yet, let them cook vegetarian meals for the whole family.

Time Tip

Most supermarkets now offer a wide selection of ready-made alternatives to meat, such as veggie hot dogs, deli slices, burgers and ground meat replacements.

Eleven

It's Snack Time

The Snack Monster Lives in All of Us

Most of us love to snack, and we are doing it more and more – often two to three times per day – with afternoons and evenings being the most popular snacking times. We snack on the road; we snack at our desks; we snack in our homes – we are a nation of snackers.

Six Super Reasons to Say Yes to Snacking

1. Snacks Bring Nutrition into a Busy Lifestyle

Whether you eat in your car as you race to your next meeting, or at your desk because time doesn't permit a more leisurely lunch, snacking is an efficient and easy way to make sure that you meet your nutritional needs.

2. Snacks Are a Great Way to Fill in the Gaps

Snacking is the perfect way to eat more of the foods you sometimes miss out on, like fruits and vegetables or milk products. It's the perfect way to fill the gaps in a less than perfect day.

3. Energize Yourself

Going long periods of time without eating is not a good idea. Ideally, you should never go more than about 4 hours without eating something (I rarely go more than 3). Research shows that meal skippers get less work done and make decisions more slowly. Research also shows that regular snacking helps regulate blood sugar levels. Fewer dips in blood sugar levels mean fewer dips in energy levels. More snacks mean more energy. It all makes such good sense.

4. Kids Were Built to Snack

Although regular snacking is important for adults, it's absolutely essential for children. Children have high calorie and nutrient needs relative to their size. They also have small stomachs. Few children can sit down to a large meal and comfortably finish it off. Regular snacks can help provide some of the nutrition that a growing child needs but may not get at mealtime.

5. Healthy for Your Heart

According to a University of Toronto study, eating 6 mini-meals per day, rather than 3 larger meals, is good for your heart. The people in this study who followed a frequent meal plan reduced the level of cholesterol in their blood by 8%, which translates into a potential 16% reduction in heart attack risk. Quite amazing, when you think it wasn't what they ate, but when they ate it, that made the difference.

6. Waistline Management

Have you ever been so hungry that when you finally got your hands on some food you gobbled up everything in sight? Out-of-control hunger is a calorie disaster just waiting to happen. It's far easier to manage your appetite when you eat frequent small meals.

Three Reasons to Approach Snacking with Caution

1. You Are What You Eat

Snacking is only as good as the snacks you choose. If most of your snacks belong in the nutritional wasteland category (high fat, low fibre, no vitamins or minerals), snacking may do you more harm than good.

2. Waistline Expansion

Just as regular snacking can help control appetite and help manage your waistline, too much snacking can cause the waistline to expand. What's more, it's easy to overeat when you snack. You can't eat 3 large meals every day and then add snacks on top. All meals should be smaller, with snacks filling in the gaps.

3. Non-Hunger Eating

Up to 50% of snacking occurs when people are bored, not hungry. When it comes to snacking, we need to be conscious fuelers, not mindless consumers. We need to be aware of what we're eating and how much. Most importantly, we should eat only when we're hungry.

The Bronze, Silver and Gold Snacking Lists

Contrary to popular belief, the perfect snack is not just low in fat. Ideally it should also be high in nutrition and, if possible, no slouch when it comes to fibre. To guide you in your snacking decisions I have devised three lists of snacking options. Gold and silver snacks, which are more nutritious, should be consumed on a regular basis. Bronze snacks, which are primarily low in fat, but not as nutritious, should be consumed less often.

The Bronze List of Snacks

The Bronze snacks are primarily low in fat, but not nutritional power hitters. They can be improved by combining them with something from the gold or silver list.

Baked Potato Chips   Potato chips are Canadians' number one snack food. We eat them by the truckload. Unfortunately, with every handful of potato chips comes a handful of fat. Fortunately, today's fat-conscious consumer can buy potato chips that have been baked rather than fried. SnackWells Potato Thins, Bitelife Potato Crisps and Dare Wise Cracks are just a few of the brands currently available. Although some argue they don't taste like the real thing, they're a pretty good substitute. By the way, beware of potato chips, like "multigrain" chips, that sound healthy but are not. Many of these healthy-sounding snacks are still deep-fried and are thus a haven for fat grams. When in doubt, check the label. Look for snacks that contain 3 grams of fat per serving or less.

Baked Tortilla Chips   Just as baked potato chips have started to grow in popularity, so have baked tortilla chips, like Baked Tostitos. The great thing about these snacks is that when you dip them in salsa (which is always a low-fat, healthy dipping option), the taste is

The Bronze List Of Snacks
in alphabetical order

Baked potato chips
Baked tortilla chips
Crackers
Granola/cereal bars
Popcorn
Pretzels
Rice cakes

superb. Pita Puffs, made from baked pita bread, are another delicious low-fat snack.

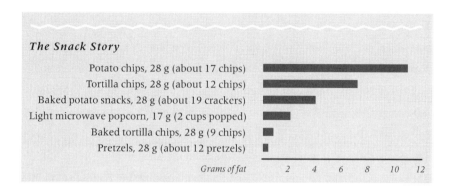

The Snack Story

	Grams of fat
Potato chips, 28 g (about 17 chips)	
Tortilla chips, 28 g (about 12 chips)	
Baked potato snacks, 28 g (about 19 crackers)	
Light microwave popcorn, 17 g (2 cups popped)	
Baked tortilla chips, 28 g (9 chips)	
Pretzels, 28 g (about 12 pretzels)	

Crackers When it comes to crackers, be aware of three things when reading labels. First, don't be fooled by healthy sounding names – most crackers offer little in the way of nutrition or fibre. Second, look for lower-fat varieties (Air Crisps get top marks for taste). Third, choose whole grain crackers if possible. To make certain, check that whole wheat flour is listed first on the ingredient list. Some of the best low-fat, high-fibre choices are the crispbreads that come under brand names like Wasa and Ryvita. Unfortunately, their taste does not appeal to all people ("cardboard" is a term frequently used).

Granola/Cereal Bars These bars have hit the market with a vengeance. People take them to work in their briefcases. Kids pack them in their lunch boxes. Although these snacks are a much better choice than a chocolate bar, they are increasingly taking the place of much healthier options, such as a piece of fruit or a container of yogurt. When you buy these snacks, check that rolled oats or whole wheat is first on the ingredient list and that there is at least 1 gram of fibre per bar. Better yet, try out the recipe on p.168 for Apple Breakfast Bars for even more nutrition.

Popcorn If I had to pick my favourite snack in the bronze category, it would be popcorn. There are three things I like about popcorn. First, although popcorn can't be considered a high flyer from a nutritional point of view, it is a good source of fibre. Second, popcorn leaves people feeling fuller much longer than many of its snack food rivals. Third, and most important, popcorn tastes great. Air-popped popcorn is the low-fat all-star, while light microwave popcorn wins in terms of convenience. Don't make the mistake of drowning your popcorn in butter. A better alternative is to give it a quick spritz with a nonstick vegetable oil spray, and then sprinkle on your favourite herbs and spices. My daughter likes her popcorn with a light dusting of sugar and cinnamon. Other tasty options include Parmesan cheese, onion salt or garlic powder. Try to steer clear of the popcorn served in most movie theatres. Even without added butter, it is much higher in fat than the kind you make at home.

Pretzels   Many a snack bowl previously dedicated to potato chips now holds only pretzels. Pretzels, without question, are very low in fat. They are, however, king of the snack heap when it comes to salt. A small handful of pretzels can contain up to 500 mg of the stuff (2,400 mg of salt is the recommended daily limit). A diet high in salt is associated with an increased risk of high blood pressure, among other things. Thus, you have three options: you can buy unsalted pretzels (too boring for most); you can buy regular pretzels and scrape off some of the salt as you eat them (my sister does this), or you can eat them in moderation just as they are.

Rice Cakes   Rice cakes are not what they used to be (boring and bland). Today they come in a wide variety of sizes and flavours, such as caramel corn, white cheddar or apple cinnamon. Most are made from a combination of corn (with the germ removed) and whole grain brown rice. They are much lower in salt than snack foods like potato chips, popcorn and pretzels. For more nutrition, eat them with something from the gold category, like a slice of melted low-fat cheese.

The Silver List of Snacks

The Silver snacks include the middle-of-the-road snacking options. These snacks are not the best of the best, and yet they are pretty darn good.

Frozen Yogurt   Low-fat frozen yogurt has all the goodness of milk in a less concentrated form. You can find it in airports, in malls, and in many fast-food outlets. Frozen yogurt bars are also widely available. Look for low-fat varieties.

Muffins   Most muffins from your local doughnut or muffin shop are very high in fat. Your best bet is to make a big batch of healthy muffins from scratch (see recipes on p.169–170) and freeze them. Grab one and let it thaw or pop it in the microwave when you need a snack.

Whole Grain Breads   There are two things you can do to maximize the nutritional contribution of breads. First, pick whole grains whenever possible. Whole wheat bagels, whole wheat pita bread and whole wheat English muffins are now widely available. Second, rather than topping your bread with butter or margarine, combine it with something from the gold category. Melt cheese on it; have a glass of milk with your bagel; make a sandwich to go.

The Gold List of Snacks

The Gold snacks provide many of the nutrients essential for good health. With the exception of milk products, these snacks are also a good source of fibre.

Bean Dips   Bean dips such as hummus (chickpea dip) are great served with wedges of whole wheat pita bread, a trayful of veggies or some baked tortilla chips. While you can make a bean dip from scratch, most stores now carry a wide selection of ready-made options.

The Silver List of Snacks
in alphabetical order

Frozen yogurt
Muffins (low-fat, high-fibre)
Whole grain breads (bagels,
English muffins, rolls)

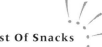

The Gold List Of Snacks
in alphabetical order

Bean dips (like hummus)
Cereal
Cheese (low-fat)
Fruit
Instant bean soup
Milk
Nuts and peanut butter
  (in moderation)
Small sandwich
Vegetables
Yogurt

Cereal   I'm a cereal fanatic. The goodness of cereal combined with the goodness of milk makes a powerful combination. Some people like cereal as a bedtime snack, others as an afternoon filler. Kids tend to like it anytime. Whenever possible, choose the high-fibre cereals.

Cheese   Although low-fat cheese is recommended (especially for adults), regular cheese is still an option when consumed in small quantities. Serve cheese with crackers. Melt it on a bagel. Eat it on its own. And remember, when it comes to taste, low-fat cheeses have improved by leaps and bounds.

Fruit   After all the fuss I've made about fruits and vegetables, you had to know fruit would be on the list. If you have trouble meeting your daily fruit or vegetable quota, snacking can make all the difference. And many fruits are so easily portable.

Instant Bean Soup   Just add hot water and serve: bean soup can be that easy. There are lots of instant varieties to choose from but the best choices are the lower-fat, salt-reduced ones.

Milk   A glass of milk (ideally 1% or skim) offers a whole lot of nutrition in the middle of a busy day. Both chocolate milk and hot chocolate (made with milk, not water) are wonderful, tasty options. A café au lait or a caffe latte at your local coffee shop can also fit the bill.

Nuts and Peanut Butter (in moderation)   Both nuts and peanut butter are highly nutritious, but also high in fat. Fortunately, they contain primarily heart-healthy fats. As long as you balance your fat intake over the rest of the day, and eat these foods in moderation, they can easily fit into a healthy diet. Peanut butter is particularly popular with children and should not be restricted due to the fat it contains.

Small Sandwich   A small sandwich served on whole grain bread with lean meat, such as turkey, chicken, ham or roast beef, makes a deli-

---

The Eight Most Portable Fruit Options

Apples

Bananas

Canned fruit cups

Clementines (and other easy-to-peel citrus fruits like tangerines)

Dried fruit (apples, apricots, dates, pears, prunes, raisins)

Fruit juice (in moderation)

Fruit paks (like applesauce)

Grapes

cious mini-meal. Water-packed tuna and salmon with light mayonnaise are also great sandwich fillers.

Vegetables The most portable way to eat vegetables is as juice. Vegetable juice is easy to carry and easy to stash in a briefcase or car. Because it is high in salt, consume it in moderation. Veggies and dip are another popular snacking option. And you don't have to cut up 5 different types of vegetables to make it worthwhile. A couple of sliced carrots will do the trick nicely. Low-fat salad dressing is an easy dipping option.

Yogurt Yogurt is a portable, great-tasting, nutrient-rich snack. Choose brands that contain less than 2% M.F. Another option, similar to yogurt but milder in taste, is fresh cheese (soft, unripened cheese you can eat with a spoon).

A Word about Candy

Many people choose ju-jubes, Gummi Bears, and licorice as low-fat snacks. The upside of these snacks is that they can help tackle cravings for something more decadent. The downside is that they provide mostly empty calories, in other words nothing of significance in the way of vitamins or minerals. So go ahead and enjoy candy – but only once in a while.

In a Nutshell...

Snacks are great for helping you meet your nutritional needs, filling in the gaps, and keeping your energy levels high. They can help keep your appetite in check, are healthy for your heart, and are essential for kids. When choosing snacks, look for those that are low in fat, make a valuable contribution on the nutritional front and are a good source of fibre.

Twelve

Desserts Make Life More Fun!

"The Urge To Splurge"– Three Ways to Handle It

Most of us love desserts, but we also realize that if we eat chocolate cake morning, noon and night, not only will our waistlines expand, we won't have room left for more nutritious foods. Does this mean we have to give up desserts entirely? Absolutely not! Here are three simple ways to handle the urge to splurge.

1. The 80/20 Rule

The 80/20 rule states that if you eat healthy foods 80% of the time, it's okay to indulge yourself the other 20% of the time. The key is to pick something you really like and to take the time to savour each and every bite. Don't rush because you feel guilty. Close your eyes, smell the food. Bite into it slowly. Notice all the different flavours, the textures, the way it feels going down your throat. Make it last. Try this

"Never eat more than you can lift."
Miss Piggy

"The best way to lose weight is to watch your food – just watch it, don't eat it."

Edward Koch

Clear the Confusion
Moderation doesn't mean giving up foods you enjoy, it means having smaller amounts less often.

with all your meals, not just dessert. You'll be surprised how much more enjoyable eating can be.

2. Fight Chocolate with Chocolate

For many people, especially women it seems, the number one craving is for chocolate. Nothing else will do. Eating an apple or an orange just isn't an option. It's chocolate you crave and it's chocolate you must have. But, the problem with chocolate is its relatively high fat and calorie content. The average chocolate bar contains about 20 grams of fat and 300 calories. Fortunately, you have three options when a chocolate craving strikes. Option 1 – have a small piece of the real thing. Option 2 – have a fat-reduced chocolate bar, such as Sweet Escapes by Hershey (have only one, ideally the snack size). Option 3 – have an alternative, low-fat chocolate fix.

The Dessert Story

	Grams of fat
Decadent Dessert Choices	
Carrot cake (1 slice)	31
Cheesecake (1 slice)	28
Pecan pie (1 slice)	24
Premium ice cream	
(125 mL/$\frac{1}{2}$ cup)	20
Chocolate bar (60g/2 oz)	19
Apple pie	17
Lower-Fat Dessert Choices	
Light apple crisp	6.0
Low-fat frozen yogurt	
(125 mL/$\frac{1}{2}$ cup)	2.2
Low-fat cookies (2)	2.1
Rice Krispies squares	
(1 square)	2.0
Angelfood cake	.2
Fruit salad (250 mL/ 1 cup)	.2

Please note: When it comes to desserts, low-fat does not mean low-calorie! All desserts, even the low-fat ones, should be consumed in moderation. Calories still count.

Top Ten Low-Fat Chocolate Fixes
in alphabetical order

1. Chocolate caramels/Tootsie Rolls
2. Chocolate chip bagel
3. Chocolate flavoured coffee
4. Hot chocolate (made with 1% or skim milk)
5. Low-fat Fudgsicle
6. Low-fat chocolate pudding
7. Low-fat chocolate chip muffin
8. Low-fat chocolate cookie
9. Low-fat chocolate brownie
10. Low-fat chocolate Pop Tart

Please note:
1. Not everything on the low-fat Chocolate Fix list is created equal when it comes to calories. For example, although 1 chocolate caramel is fairly innocent, a chocolate Pop Tart or brownie can contribute significantly to your caloric intake. As always, proceed with caution. Your waistline will thank you for it.
2. This philosophy of fighting chocolate with chocolate also applies to other food cravings. If your craving is for something salty like potato chips, find a reasonable salty but low-fat substitute like baked potato chips or pretzels. If its something sweet that calls your name, a slice of raisin toast, a piece of fruit, or even some low-fat candy (like jelly beans) might do the trick.

> **News Flash: Dietitians Eat Chocolate** In a recent survey of more than a thousand Canadian dietitians, 97% said they eat chocolate and candy themselves (I was one of them and proud of it).

3. Ride the Wave

Don't give in every time you experience the urge to splurge. Research from the University of Washington shows that cravings follow a wave pattern. Cravings start and escalate, but then peak and subside. Successful dieters agree. In a recent study, when asked what was the best way to handle food cravings, their most common reply was "wait it out."

The Winners of the Healthy Dessert Competition

If you like to indulge on a more regular basis, let me tell you about the two winners of the Healthy Dessert Competition. These desserts meet three criteria – they taste great, they're low in fat, and they're nutritious.

1. Fabulous Frozen Yogurt

Frozen yogurt is fabulous. I always keep a tub of low-fat frozen yogurt in my freezer. Frozen yogurt contains many of the wonderful nutrients found in a glass of milk – like protein, riboflavin and calcium – only in a less concentrated form. Frozen yogurt also tastes great and comes in a variety of flavours. What's more, there are so many fun and tasty ways to serve it! Here are three delicious ways to serve frozen yogurt:

1. *All by Itself* Indulge in the explosion of flavour options: Raspberry Rendezvous, Orange Tango, Strawberry Duet, Chocolate Thunder and Vanilla Royale.
2. *As a Sundae* My daughter loves frozen yogurt sundaes. We start with low-fat vanilla frozen yogurt. We add some sliced

Super Nutrition Tip
Most frozen yogurts contains more nutrition and significantly less fat than ice cream.

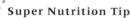

bananas, then drizzle chocolate or strawberry syrup on top, and add a few sprinkles for extra appeal. It sounds decadent, but it's not – especially since most instant chocolate and strawberry syrups contain less than 1 gram of fat per tablespoon (15 mL).

3. *A Fruit and Frozen Yogurt Combo*   Frozen yogurt and fruit is a wonderful and nutritious combination, particularly for those people who think fruit served on its own is simply too boring. The fruit can be fresh, canned, or even frozen. Try heating frozen raspberries or blueberries in the microwave and drizzle them on top for a special treat.

2. Fantastic Fruit

Fruit satisfies the craving for something sweet at the end of the meal. It's also low in fat and loaded with valuable vitamins, minerals, phytochemicals and more. There's only one problem. Some people think it lacks excitement. That's probably because they haven't tried any of the suggestions listed below:

1. *Sensational Strawberries*   Mix strawberries with a dash of balsamic vinegar and a touch of sugar. Absolutely delicious.

2. *Peaches Royale*   Spoon low-fat or light sour cream into fresh or canned peach halves. Sprinkle with brown sugar. Place under the broiler until sugar caramelizes. A peach of a treat.

3. *Banana Broiler*   Drizzle sliced bananas with lemon juice, brown sugar and a touch of shredded coconut. Place under broiler until the bananas are golden brown and tender. Sweet and succulent.

4. *Crepe Supreme*   Mix diced fruit, like peaches, pears or mangoes, with plain yogurt. Place inside a store-bought crepe. Drizzle with chocolate syrup. Truly decadent.

5. *Frozen Fruit Skewers*   Arrange kiwi wedges, whole strawberries and grapes on wooden skewers. Put in the freezer. When

frozen, they are ready for eating. Cool and refreshing on a hot day.

6. *Applesauce Divine*   Sprinkle unsweetened applesauce with brown sugar, cinnamon and a dash of nutmeg. Heat in the microwave for less than 1 minute. For kids, add sprinkles. Tasty and fun.

7. *Dip 'n' Dunk Strawberries*   Dip strawberries in light sour cream, then in brown sugar. Sweet and satisfying.

8. *Baked Apple Slices*   Toss peeled apple wedges in a touch of flour, sugar and cinnamon. Use vegetable oil spray to grease baking sheet. Spread apples on sheet and bake in oven (450 F/230 C) for 15 to 20 minutes or until golden brown and tender. A heavenly treat.

9. *Fruit Salad Sensation*   Mix 3 cups (750 mL) chopped fresh fruit with 1 cup (250 mL) low-fat sour cream, 1 tablespoon (15 mL)honey or maple syrup, and 1 teaspoon (5 mL) grated orange peel. Cover and refrigerate for 1 hour before eating. Always a hit.

10. *Pineapple Griller*   Grill pineapple rings on the barbecue until golden brown. The sugar in the pineapple will caramelize during cooking. So juicy and sweet.

A Word about Cookies

Although cookies can't compare to frozen yogurt or fruit in nutritional value, they are lower in both fat and calories than most other desserts (like pies, cakes and ice cream). This advantage, however, applies only if you eat cookies in a reasonable fashion. Unfortunately, many of us suffer from the "cookie monster" syndrome. We start with good intentions, but before you know it, 2 cookies turn into 4, 4 cookies turn into 8, and in mere minutes an entire bagful has been devoured. To fight the cookie monster, try to keep the number 2 uppermost in your mind. Two Oreo cookies, for example, translates into 4.3 grams of fat and 100 calories. Ten Oreo cookies, on the other hand, contain almost 22 grams of fat and 500 calories. That's quite a difference (and remember, most low-fat cookies, such as SnackWells or Fig Newtons, contain the same amount of calories as their higher-fat counterparts). So go ahead and have your 2 cookies. Just don't let the Cookie Monster talk you into any more.

In a Nutshell...

Healthful eating means enjoying all foods, including desserts. Choose more often those desserts, like low-fat frozen yogurt and fruit, that not only taste great, but also provide good nutrition. And don't forget, when it comes to dessert, calories still count.

The Beverage Story

Water – The Forgotten Nutrient

Water – You've Gotta Have It

The importance of water is best illustrated by the fact that we can live for several weeks without food, but only a few days without water. The human body is made up of about 60 to 70% water (an incredible 40 litres of water in the average adult). Name almost any major function of the human body, and water plays a starring role. Water makes it possible to digest food and absorb all its wonderful nutrients. Water acts as the body's natural air-conditioning system; the loss of water through perspiration cools the body and prevents it from overheating. In fact, every living cell in our bodies depends on water to carry out its essential functions.

Clear the Confusion
Contrary to popular belief, the mineral content of most mineral waters is not enough to significantly influence your nutritional status.

Clear the Confusion
Why are people who are trying to lose weight often told to drink 8 glasses of water per day? Although water does not have any magic powers when it comes to fat-burning, a study from the University of Toronto suggests that a couple of glasses before a meal helps to keep your appetite in check. Bottoms up.

Hydration Tip
If you feel thirsty, drink. Thirst is your body's way of telling you the water level is getting too low and it's time to visit the water cooler. The only drawback to this mechanism is that it loses its sensitivity as we age – another reason that the 8-a-day guideline makes good sense.

Hydration Tip
If you are physically active, pregnant, or ill, it's a good idea to increase your water intake beyond the 8-a-day guideline.

Hydration Tip
To prevent dehydration when flying, drink 1 glass of water for every hour in flight.

Eight Glasses a Day

So what's the deal on the often-heard recommendation that we drink 8 glasses of water a day? Replacement is the name of the game. All day long we lose water – as we breathe, when we perspire, each time we make a trip to the toilet. The average person loses about 2 to 3 litres per day. For optimal health and well-being, that water must be replaced. Thus, the "8-a-day" rule comes into play.

Your "Eight-a-day" Quota – Four Tips to Figuring Out Your Intake

If you can't remember the last time you drank 8 glasses of water in one day, not to worry. It's much easier to meet your water quota than most people think. Here are some tips.

1. Liquids of All Kinds

With the exception of coffee, tea and alcohol, all fluids count towards your daily water quota, including milk, juice, soft drinks and soup.

2. Coffee and Tea

Although both coffee and tea are diuretics, which means that they increase water loss, they still contribute to your water intake. The key is to count every 3 cups of coffee or tea as only 2 cups of fluid.

3. Alcohol

Alcohol, as most people know, is extremely dehydrating. On the morning after a night of overindulgence this becomes most evident. That's why for every glass of wine, bottle of beer or mixed drink you consume you need to drink an extra glass of water over and above your 8-a-day quota.

4. Solids

Fruits and vegetables also make a valuable contribution on the water front. Don't expect to calculate how much water they contribute. Just feel good knowing they are helping you in your daily quest for full hydration.

What to Drink When You're Active

Generally speaking, the more you move around, the more water you require. For most people, drinking 1 to 2 glasses of water 1 hour prior to being active will compensate for any water lost through perspiration. If your exercise is of a more strenuous nature, drink small quantities of water regularly throughout your workout. Sports drinks, which contain primarily simple sugars, need be consumed only if you are exercising quite strenuously for longer than 1 hour or in conditions of extreme heat or humidity.

Is Our Tap Water Safe to Drink?

Is our water safe to drink? This is by no means an easy question to answer. On one hand, Canada has some of the best drinking-water treatment facilities in the world. Water from virtually any source (even the most polluted) can be made suitable for drinking by water treatment, which includes both the filtering and disinfection of water. Municipal water supplies are tested regularly for the presence of harmful bacteria, as well as for several hundred chemicals. Technology has been developed to the point that scientists are able to detect the presence of chemicals at extremely low levels – parts per trillion or even parts per quadrillion. Major steps have been taken to reduce the quantity of all potentially harmful substances, such as aluminum and trihalomethanes (by-products as a result of disinfection with chlorine). What this means is that, overall, the Canadian water supply is pretty darn safe.

Hydration Tip
One of the easiest ways to tell if you're well hydrated is by the colour of your urine. If your urine is pale yellow or clear, you're in great shape. If your urine is deep yellow, then it's time to drink up. By the way, this test is not valid upon waking each morning.

Hydration Tip
If you work in an office, one of the easiest ways to up your water intake is to place a large pitcher of water on your desk first thing in the morning. Once it's there and ready to pour, you'll find it disappears with no effort at all. Not only will you stay hydrated, the few extra trips to the bathroom will give your legs a stretch.

Hydration Tip
One of the hidden dangers of tap water is lead, which can leach in when water flows through lead pipes that connect water mains to home plumbing. It's a good idea to let the water run for a minute or two (until it runs cold) before drinking it. This caution applies primarily to older homes, and to times when water sits in the pipes for more than 5 hours (for example, overnight).

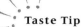

Taste Tip
If the taste and odour of the chlorine found in tap water has you buying bottled water, there is a simple solution. Fill a jug with tap water and leave it in the fridge overnight. The chlorine will dissipate, leaving you with better-tasting water.

Clear the Confusion
Some groups believe that fluoride in water may be dangerous to health. Study after study, however, has failed to support this belief. The main reason for adding fluoride to our drinking water is to enhance our dental health. Fluoride in drinking water can reduce cavities by 40 to 50%, particularly among children. Most bottled water does not contain fluoride.

The Bottled Water versus Tap Water Debate

Although some people prefer the taste of bottled water, it is not necessarily safer to drink. The safety of any water depends on where it comes from, the type of treatment used to ensure its safety, and the testing of the final product. Generally speaking, both municipal water supplies (tap water) and bottled water supplies are carefully monitored and tested to ensure high quality and safety.

The Pitfall of Home Water Treatment Systems

Water treatment systems you can use at home range from simple carafe type filters, like Brita water filters, to much more expensive and complex systems that attach directly to your water supply. Generally speaking, the larger the filter and the longer the contact time, the more effectively it will remove substances such as lead from your water. Here's the problem. You must remember to change the filter frequently. If filters are not changed regularly, they can become a breeding ground for bacteria and can actually make the water unsafe to drink. If you change the filters regularly, however, these devices can be effective in improving the quality of your water.

News Flash: Water Safety   Never drink water directly from lakes or streams. Parasites that can cause illness, such as cryptosporidium and giardia, may be present in even the most pristine-looking waters. These parasites are killed when water is boiled for at least 1 minute.

In a Nutshell...

For good health and proper hydration, drink 8 glasses of water or other fluids each day. Overall, both tap water and bottled water can be considered safe to drink.

Hooked on Caffeine – How Much Is Too Much?

The Number One Drug of Choice

As you sip your morning coffee you may not think of caffeine as a drug, but it is. Millions of people around the world wake up in the morning and feel better once they've had their morning brew. That's because caffeine stimulates our central nervous system and makes us feel more awake and alert.

The Good News about Caffeine

If you thought I was going to give you a long list of reasons why you should bid farewell to your daily brew, you are mistaken. In fact, the more studies one looks at, the more evident it becomes that for most people moderate amounts of coffee and caffeine have no adverse effects on health. For example, contrary to popular belief, coffee does not increase the risk of heart disease. In the Nurses' Health Study, even women who drank 6 or more cups of coffee a day faced no higher risk. As for cancer, studies have failed to show a link between coffee or caffeine intake and cancer incidence. Having said all that, there are a few exceptions to the rule. Children and mothers-to-be should approach caffeine with caution.

News Flash: Coffee In Moderation   Health Canada defines a moderate caffeine intake as 400 to 450 mg per day or about 3 cups of coffee per day. For some people, too much caffeine can lead to "coffee nerves," which are characterized by insomnia, headaches, irritability and nervousness.

Coffee Trivia
Within 30 to 60 minutes of drinking a cup of coffee, caffeine reaches its peak concentration level in our bloodstream and we feel its maximum effects. Typically, it takes 4 to 6 hours for its effects to wear off completely.

Clear the Confusion
Back in the 1970s, the headlines warned that decaffeinated coffee was not safe to drink because of its cancer-causing potential. Those concerns arose primarily because of one solvent, trichlorethylene, used to extract the caffeine. The new solvents have a clean bill of health. In addition, residual solvent (small traces of solvent left in decaffeinated products) is legally restricted in Canada to very low levels to ensure safe drinking for all.

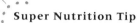

Super Nutrition Tip
Turn your coffee into a nutritional superstar, drink it *au lait* or *latte* more often. You get the pleasure of coffee with all the goodness of milk – the calcium, vitamin D and riboflavin. For less fat, use skim or 1% milk.

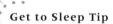

Get to Sleep Tip
If you have trouble falling asleep, you may want to avoid caffeine in the latter parts of the day. Not only can caffeine delay the onset of sleep, but it can also interfere with rapid eye movement (REM) sleep, the stage when people dream.

Caffeine And Breastfeeding
Breastfeeding mothers who love a sleeping baby (and who doesn't?) should moderate their intake of caffeine. Caffeine in breast milk may keep baby awake.

News Flash: Mega Coffee   The amount of caffeine in coffee can vary quite considerably depending on the amount of coffee used to make the brew and the size of the cup. The mega coffees available at some coffee houses contain a whopping 550 mg per serving (a regular size coffee contains about 140 mg).

Kids and Caffeine

Because caffeine has a stronger effect on smaller bodies, children's intake of caffeine is of particular concern. The Framingham Children's Study found that kids get about 55% of their caffeine from soft drinks, with another 38% from chocolate. For a small child, 1 can of cola can have the same effect as 2 to 4 cups of coffee in an adult. Therefore, if your kids drink pop, which ideally should be on an occasional basis rather than a regular basis (pop tends to replace more nutritious drinks like milk), be sure to choose those brands that are caffeine-free. Chocolate products, like chocolate bars, chocolate milk or even chocolate chip cookies are not of concern as long as these foods are consumed in reasonable quantities.

Baby and Java Don't Jive

Over the years the effects of caffeine on pregnancy have been a most controversial issue. One study says no problem, the next study says watch out. Currently, Health Canada maintains that 400 to 450 mg of caffeine per day should not increase the risk of adverse effects on pregnancy or the fetus. Some current studies suggest, however, that reducing caffeine even further may be beneficial. For example, in 1993, the American Medical Association published a major study that found that pregnant women who drank from 1.5 to 3 cups of coffee per day doubled their risk of miscarriage. Women who drank more than 3 cups tripled their risk. These findings are consistent with a 1996 Yale University study, which found twice as great a miscarriage risk in those women who consumed more than 300 mg of caffeine per day.

Some studies have also shown that caffeine can inhibit the ability to conceive.

Bottom line: when it comes to pregnancy, why take chances? Pregnant women should limit their caffeine intake to a minimum or avoid it altogether.

News Flash: Heartburn And Ulcer   If you suffer from stomach ulcers or heartburn, you may want to watch your coffee intake, whether regular or decaf. Coffee stimulates the flow of stomach acid and thus potentially irritates the stomach lining and ulcers. Coffee also relaxes the sphincter at the end of the esophagus, increasing the risk of heartburn in some people.

News Flash: Stop The Headache   If 1 to 2 aspirin tablets don't relieve your headache, a cup of coffee along with them might be just the prescription you need. A little caffeine can boost the effectiveness of aspirin, acetaminophen and other pain relievers by up to 40%.

The Withdrawal Reality

Research from Johns Hopkins University indicates that people who drink even 1 or 2 cups of coffee or tea a day can suffer from withdrawal when they miss their daily dose. Headaches, fatigue, depression and anxiety are all symptoms of caffeine withdrawal. Some anesthesiologists even suggest using intravenous caffeine to help prevent coffee and cola drinkers from enduring withdrawal headaches after surgery.

Bottom line: if you want to cut back on caffeine, do so gradually (the technical term is "caffeine fading"). Most people report good success by cutting down at the rate of about half a cup per day.

In a Nutshell...

For most people, moderate amounts of coffee and caffeine have no adverse effects on health. Children and mothers-to-be, however, should approach caffeine with caution.

Caffeine Content

Reminder: A moderate amount is 400–450 mg/day

	mg
Coffee: per 175 mL cup/6 oz	
Coffee, drip	110–180
Coffee, instant	60–90
Coffee, decaffeinated	2–6
Coffee, espresso	
(60 mL/2 oz)	90–110
Tea: per 175 mL cup/6oz	
Iced tea	25–80
Weak tea	20–45
Strong tea	70–110
Chocolate:	
Chocolate milk	
(250 mL/1 cup)	8–10
Dark chocolate bar	
(56 g/2 oz)	40–50
Milk chocolate bar	
(56 g/2 oz)	10–20
Chocolate cake	
(1 slice)	20–30
Soft Drinks: 350 mL/12 oz	
Colas	35–45

Please note: Caffeine is also found in some headache and cold relief medications.

Move Over Coffee, Here Comes Tea

Time to Trade in the Coffee Mug for a Cup of Tea

Although health experts have given moderate coffee drinkers the green light, may I suggest that you consider trading in your coffee mug for a cup of tea? Although your morning coffee won't do you any harm, why not switch to a beverage that could potentially enhance your overall health by reducing your risk of both heart disease and cancer?

Tea Trivia
There are three main types of tea – green, black, and oolong. They all come from the same source, the *Camellia sinensis* bush. However, each one is processed in a different manner. Almost 90% of the tea consumed in Canada is black, while people in Asia prefer green or oolong tea.

News Flash: Tea Discovery It is believed that tea was discovered by a Chinese emperor when a tea leaf accidentally fell into the bowl of hot water he was drinking.

Health Benefits of Tea

More and more research is looking at polyphenols, or more specifically, flavonoids and catechins, a class of phytochemicals found in tea. Scientists believe that these polyphenols function much like antioxidants in our bodies. By putting cell-damaging free radicals out of business, they reduce the risk of both heart disease and cancer. When a University of Minnesota study analyzed the tea drinking habits of more than 35,000 women over an 8-year period, it found that women who drank 2 or more cups of tea a day had a significantly lower risk of certain types of cancer. A recent Dutch study of over 500 men found a 73% lower risk of stroke in those men whose diets were richest in flavonoids, the majority of which came from tea.

> **News Flash: Iced Tea Is Born**   Iced tea was born at the 1904
> World's Fair in St. Louis. An Englishman, Richard Blechynden, was
> trying unsuccessfully to promote tea at the fair, but the sweltering
> Missouri heat did little to attract patrons. Once he added ice cubes,
> the crowds loved the new brew.

Tea Trivia
Tipping as a response to proper
service started in the tea gardens of
England. Small locked wooden boxes
were placed throughout the gardens.
Inscribed on each were the letters
T.I.P.S. which stood for "To Insure
Prompt Service." If a guest wished
the waiter to hurry (and so ensure the
tea arrived hot from the often distant
kitchen), he or she dropped a coin
into the box.

Is Green Tea Better for You ?

Contrary to popular belief, you don't have to switch to green tea to
experience the many health-enhancing benefits of tea drinking.
Research shows promising results with both black tea and green tea.
Decaffeinated tea (not the herbal types) also contains health-enhancing polyphenols.

What about Iced Tea?

Little research has been done into the health benefits of iced tea.
Researchers speculate that those iced teas that contain a significant
amount of tea (not just sugar and water), also contain a decent quantity of health-enhancing polyphenols. Unfortunately, manufacturers
don't indicate the tea content on the label.

> **News Flash: Iced Tea Sugar Alert**   If you like to chill out with a
> long, cool glass of iced tea on a hot summer's day, beware. Many
> sweetened iced teas, like Snapple or Arizona, contain a whopping
> 15 to 16 teaspoons of sugar per bottle (600 mL/20 oz serving).

How Much Tea Do You Need to Drink ?

How much tea do you need to drink to experience its potential health-
enhancing benefits? Current studies indicate that disease risk reduction is possible with as little as 2 cups of tea a day, while even greater
benefits may be experienced by heavier tea drinkers (up to 5 cups per
day). I suggest you think of tea as just one more healthy addition to

the phytochemical-containing family of fruits, vegetables and whole grains.

What about Herbal Teas?

A herbal tea by definition does not contain any true tea leaves. Most herbal teas are made with infusions of flowers, herbs or spices. While these herbs may have health-enhancing properties of their own (which have yet to be studied in any depth), do not expect them to provide you with the same disease-reducing benefits as regular tea.

In a Nutshell...

Research indicates that tea may reduce the risk of both heart disease and cancer. Both black and green teas are effective health enhancers.

Seven Fascinating Facts about Alcohol

1. The French Paradox

When it comes to the prevention of heart attacks, "There is no other drug that is so efficient as the moderate intake of alcohol," says Serge Renaud, director of the French National Institute of Health and Medical Research.

In 1991, the CBS television show "60 Minutes" aired a segment about the "French paradox" and the possible benefits of drinking red wine. The following month, sales of red wine surged by 44% in the U.S. The French paradox goes something like this: despite a diet that includes some of the world's best cheeses, cream sauces and pastries, the French have a lower incidence of heart disease than people in many other industrialized countries, including Canada. Could it be that a few glasses of red wine are at least partly responsible? It appears so. In fact, some researchers have stated that the benefits of wine drinking in moderation are so great that its alcoholic content might be better defined as a nutrient than a drug.

2. Alcohol and Heart Health

Studies consistently show that drinking moderate amounts of alcoholic beverages reduces the risk of heart disease. There appear to be at least two mechanisms in play. First, alcohol reduces the formation of potentially harmful blood clots. Many heart attacks and strokes are caused by blood clots forming in a partially blocked artery. Second, alcohol reduces the amount of plaque (thick, yellow, fatty deposits) that forms on the artery wall. It does this by increasing the amount of HDL or "good" cholesterol in the blood. It is HDL that removes cholesterol from the blood and takes it back to the liver for disposal. The average HDL level of drinkers is 10 to 15% higher than that of non-drinkers.

> **News Flash: Alcohol and Heart Disease**   For most people over 35 years of age, the risk of heart disease is reduced by 40 to 60% by drinking moderate amounts of alcohol.

3. Red Wine May Be Better

All alcoholic beverages will reduce the risk of heart disease. However, it appears that red wine is particularly beneficial. In addition to ethanol, which is found in all alcoholic beverages, red wine contains phytochemicals called polyphenols (similar to those found in tea). These polyphenols are thought to act as antioxidants in the body. In other words, they prevent the build-up of plaque on the artery wall by putting a stop to cell-damaging free radicals. Red wine contains about twice as many polyphenols as white wine or beer. One of the most powerful polyphenols in red wine is called resveratrol.

4. If a Little Is Good, More Is Not Always Better

"Eat bread at pleasure, drink wine by measure."

Randle Cotgrave

If one glass of wine is good for the heart, would several glasses be even better? The general consensus on the health front is that the protective effects of alcohol disappear as its intake increases. In the Harvard Physicians' Health Study of more than 22,000 male doctors, the protective effects of alcohol were evident at intakes between 2 and 6 drinks per week. Beyond that, hazards like cancer – particularly cancer of the colon – and accidents were found to cancel out the benefit and, in fact, increase the risk of cancer. In the Nurses' Health Study of more than 89,000 women, the risk of dying was 19% higher – often due to breast cancer – in heavier drinkers as compared to non-drinkers. Thus, it is recommended that men consume no more than 2 drinks and women no more than one drink on any given day.

> **News Flash: Drinking In Moderation**   "Moderate drinking" is defined as no more than 2 drinks a day for men and no more than 1 drink a day for women. Women have a higher percentage of body fat and less body water than men, leading to higher blood-alcohol concentrations when a given amount of alcohol is consumed. More than 4 drinks on any one occasion or more than 14 drinks in a week are considered by Health Canada as a risk to health and safety. One drink is equal to 12 ounces of beer, 5 ounces of wine or 1.5 ounces of 80-proof spirits. All contain about 12 grams of ethanol.

5. The Alcohol – Breast Cancer Connection

Unfortunately for women, the drinking of alcohol is a double-edged sword. On one hand, women who drink alcohol significantly reduce their risk of heart disease. In the Harvard Nurses' Health Study, for example, women who consumed between 3 and 9 drinks a week had a 40% lower risk than non-drinkers. On the other hand, women who drink alcohol are also at an increased risk for breast cancer. What's more, this increased breast cancer risk occurs at the same levels of alcohol intake that offer protection against heart disease. In the Nurses' Health Study, for example, those who consumed between 3 and 9 drinks a week were 30% more likely than non-drinkers to develop breast cancer. Scientists believe that alcohol may cause breast cancer by altering the level of hormones such as estrogen. The American Cancer Society now suggests that women who are at a high risk for breast cancer because of their family history should consider abstaining from alcohol completely. Your best bet is to consider your own personal history. And keep in mind that for women heart disease is still the number one killer.

> **News Flash: Pregnancy and Alcohol Update** At this time, the amount of alcohol that is safe during pregnancy is unclear. Consequently, the prudent choice for pregnant women or women who may become pregnant is to abstain from alcohol.

6. If You Don't Drink Now, Don't Feel You Have to Start

If you abstain from alcohol for whatever reason, there is no need to start drinking now solely to decrease your risk of heart disease. Watching your saturated fat intake, eating lots of fruits, vegetables and whole grains, and getting a regular dose of physical activity will put the odds for good health in your favour.

7. Alcohol Is a Dangerous Drug

Alcohol is both addictive and intoxicating. Alcohol and tobacco are the two most physically damaging drugs of dependence. Alcohol is a factor in a third to a half of all homicides, motor vehicle fatalities, child and spouse abuse cases, suicides, drownings and injuries from falls and fires. For these reasons many health authorities are reluctant to recommend its use, and all agree that those who use alcohol should do so in moderation.

News Flash: Alcohol and Your Waistline   With the exception of some liqueurs and mixed drinks (like coffee liqueurs made with cream, or piña coladas made with coconut milk), most alcoholic drinks are fat-free, though none are calorie-free. In addition, alcohol may slow the rate at which the body burns fat. Therefore, if you want to manage your waistline, it makes sense to manage your alcohol intake as well.

Fat and Calorie Contribution from Various Alcoholic Beverages

	Calories	Grams of fat
Beer (355 mL/12 oz)	160	0
Beer, light (355 mL/12 oz)	100	0
Wine (150 mL/5 oz)	103	0
Wine cooler (355 mL/12 oz)	215	0
Spirits (45 mL/1.5 oz) (gin, rum, vodka, whisky)	97	0
Rum and Coke (250 mL/8 oz)	180	0
Vodka and orange juice (250 mL/8 oz)	187	0
Vodka and tomato juice (250 mL/8 oz)	130	0
Piña colada (210 mL/7 oz)	525	16.9
Coffee liqueur (45 mL/1.5 oz)	160	.1
Coffee liqueur with cream (45 mL/1.5 oz)	154	7.4

In a Nutshell...

Alcohol in moderate amounts significantly reduces the risk of heart disease. Red wine appears to offer greater protection against heart disease than other alcoholic beverages. Even moderate alcohol consumption may increase the risk of breast cancer for women.

Fourteen

Pass the Sugar, Hold the Salt

Sugar: The Number One Myth Maker

Current Canadian guidelines do not tell people to avoid or reduce their sugar intake. In fact, sugar is not even mentioned. Former guidelines did recommend a reduction in sugar intake, but this advice was dropped when the bulk of scientific evidence did not support it. However, although the guidelines have changed, people's outlook on sugar has not. In fact, if there were a "Top Food Myth" award, sugar myths would be prime contenders.

> **News Flash: Sugar Calorie Surprise** Most people overestimate the number of calories in 1 teaspoon of sugar. In a recent survey the average guess was 70 calories per teaspoon. In reality, sugar contains 16 calories per teaspoon.

Top Four Sugar Myths

Myth 1. Sugar Will Make You Fat

If you eat too much sugar, will it make you fat? Yes. Then again, if you eat too much pizza, bread, cheese or spaghetti, they too could make you fat. The fact is that when you eat more calories than needed, no matter what the source, your waistline will expand. Yet sugar is no more likely to pack on the pounds than other foods. In fact, in comparison with the number one villain – fat – sugar is a fairly innocent bystander in the ongoing battle of the bulge.

Myth 2. Sugar Causes Diabetes

Yes, people who have diabetes must keep track of how much carbohydrate, including sugar, they eat as part of a carefully planned diet. Sugar does not, however, cause diabetes to occur in the first place. A family history of diabetes and obesity are the major risk factors in its development. What's more, in the past people with diabetes were advised to avoid the simple sugars like those found in their sugar bowl, or in cakes or cookies. It was believed that these simple sugars would cause a rapid rise in blood sugar and would make control of the disease more difficult. We now know that simple sugars are processed in the body in much the same way as the starch in such foods as rice, potatoes and bread. For this reason people with diabetes now focus on the total amount of carbohydrate in their diet, rather than the source.

Read the Label
If you want to figure out how many teaspoons of sugar are contained in a particular product, simply divide the grams of sugar as listed on the product label by 4 (1 teaspoon sugar equals 4 grams). For example, if a container of yogurt holds 16 grams of sugar, this equals 4 teaspoons of sugar per serving.

Read the Label
If the label says "no sugar added," it does not mean that the product does not contain sugar. It simply means that no sugars were added during processing. Canned fruit, for example, can claim to have "no sugar added" even though both the fruit and the juice contain a substantial amount of naturally occurring sugar.

News Flash: Dental Health Although sugar gets a clean bill of health when it comes to major health problems like heart disease and cancer, it is forced to plead guilty when it comes to dental decay (in other words, cavities). Sugar-containing foods that stick to your teeth, such as jelly beans and raisins, are among the worst offenders. What most people fail to realize, however, is that all carbohydrates, including starchy foods like bread, cereals and crackers, are also harmful to teeth. Happy brushing!

Myth 3. Sugar Causes Hyperactivity in Children

Parents, teachers and even some doctors believe sugar is the most common cause of hyperactive behaviour. And yet a substantial body of research has shown absolutely no link between sugar intake and hyperactivity. One of the best designed and most carefully controlled studies looked not only at normal preschool children, but also at school children described by their parents as sensitive to sugar. The children and their families followed a different diet for 3 consecutive 3-week periods. The results? Even when sugar was consumed at 6 times the typical amount, it had no effect on the children's behaviour. Other studies have confirmed this finding and have, in fact, shown that sugar – like other types of carbohydrate – can even have a calming effect. If you claim this can't be true – that you've seen your child start "bouncing off the walls" at parties where sweets are offered – well, there's more. Scientists have carefully studied the behaviour of children on special occasions, serving half of them foods containing real sugar while the other half received artificially sweetened foods. All children were equally turbulent. Researchers concluded that just being at a party is probably a good enough reason to get excited. Also, keep in mind that kids can get disruptive when they are overstimulated, overtired or have consumed too much caffeine (usually in the form of soft drinks).

Read the Label
Don't be fooled by labels on jams, jellies and kids' snacks that say "100% fruit" or "made with fruit juice." Most of these products are sweetened with fruit juice concentrate, which is basically sugar and has no fewer calories or more nutrients than regular sugar.

Clear the Confusion
Sugar does not cause low blood sugar (hypoglycemia) in healthy people. More specifically, eating sweet foods, or even pure sugar for that matter, does not cause a rapid rise in blood sugar followed by an excess surge of insulin followed by a low level of blood sugar. In reality, the human body is very good at regulating blood sugar, no matter what type or how much food is consumed.

Myth 4. Natural Sugars Are Healthier

Many people mistakenly believe that sugars that occur naturally in foods like fruit or fruit juice are healthier than sugars that are added to foods. The truth is that once eaten, all sugars are broken down to either fructose or glucose and utilized in much the same manner. They all provide calories with little in the way of other nutrients. Honey offers no nutritional advantage over white sugar. Brown sugar is no better than white. And even molasses, which is often cited as a source of iron, contains iron in a largely unabsorbable form. In other words, nutritionally speaking, sugar is sugar is sugar.

Read the Label
Fruit "canned in its own juice" contains about 1 teaspoon less sugar than regular canned fruit. When you consider the additional cost of the canned "in its own juice" kind, 1 extra teaspoon is really no big deal.

Reduce the Fat

A great way to reduce the amount of fat in your diet is with a little sugar. There's no need to add butter to sugar-glazed carrots. Sweet potatoes are delicious with a dash of maple syrup. The fat in most muffin recipes can be cut in half with a sweetened fruit purée (like applesauce). And the butter on your toast can be replaced entirely with jam.

Read the Label

If you are looking for sugar on the ingredients list, keep an eye out for "-ose" words, like glucose, fructose, sucrose and lactose, which are all different types of sugars added by manufacturers.

Sugar Makes Good Food Better

Sugar gets top honours when it increases the appeal of those foods we should eat more often. Take grapefruit, for example. Grapefruit is a wonderful source of vitamin C, and with a touch of added sugar it tastes really quite divine. The same goes for jam on whole wheat bread, maple syrup on pancakes or a sprinkle of sugar on your favourite, high-fibre cereal. All these foods provide good nutrition, and with a little added sweetness we enjoy them so much more.

Watch Out for "High-Fat" and "Sugar-Only" Foods

Although sugar gets a passing grade on the health front, there are two types of sugary foods that should be approached with caution: foods that are high in fat, such as pies, cakes and other goodies, and "sugar-only" foods, foods that are composed primarily of sugar, with little else in terms of nutritional value (hence the term "empty calories"). Soft drinks and candy are two examples of sugar-only foods. One can (355 mL/12 oz) of your average soft drink, for example, contains about 10 teaspoons of sugar, but absolutely nothing in the way of vitamins or minerals.

Sugar Substitutes – Are They Safe?

Why Use Sugar Substitutes in the First Place?

Sugar substitutes such as Nutrasweet (aspartame) and Splenda (sucralose) can reduce the number of calories you consume in a day. For example, 1 can of diet cola contains only 1 calorie, while a can of regular pop contains 150 calories. In addition, the diet cola will not harm your teeth.

But Are They Safe?

Before any sweetener is approved for market, it must meet rigorous guidelines and have undergone years of extensive testing. In addition, Health and Welfare Canada is responsible for setting an "Acceptable Daily Intake" (ADI) for each sweetener under review. The ADI is the amount of sweetener that can safely be consumed every day over a lifetime. For example, the ADI for aspartame is 40 mg per kg per day. That's a lot of aspartame. A 70-kilogram (154-pound) male would have to consume 18 cans of pop in 1 day to reach this limit (and even if he did, it still would not be considered harmful). Surveys consistently show that even the heaviest users of sugar substitutes consume quantities well below the recommended ADI levels. In other words, based on current levels of consumption, there appears to be no cause for concern when it comes to sugar substitutes.

> **News Flash: Pregnancy And Sugar Substitutes** Based on comprehensive studies in both animals and humans, both Nutrasweet and Splenda have been deemed safe for use during pregnancy.

> **News Flash: Nutrasweet Scare** Nutrasweet has been said to cause everything from headaches to nausea to mood swings to brain tumours. Years of careful scientific study, however, have failed to confirm that it can bring about adverse health effects. It is one of the most studied sugar substitutes to date and, overall, continues to get a clean bill of health.

In a Nutshell...

Sugar can be part of a healthy diet and is best used to make nutritious foods more enjoyable. With the exception of tooth decay, sugar is not considered harmful to health. Sugar substitutes are safe and can be used in moderation.

The Number One Reason to Reduce the Salt

I'm Not A Low-salt Fanatic

I enjoy a sprinkle of salt on a freshly sliced tomato. To me, an egg tastes better with a dash of salt than without. At the same time, I don't shake salt on every food I eat and I don't always use salt when cooking. I also try to limit my intake of highly salted processed foods. In other words, I use salt in moderation. And here's why...

Salt and High Blood Pressure

Hypertension, also known as high blood pressure, is a major risk factor in the development of heart disease, and is one of the most widespread health problems of the Western world. It is also the number one reason Canadians should moderate their use of salt.

The Intersalt Study

The Intersalt study, first published in 1988, looked at 10,000 people in 32 different countries and found that high blood pressure was more common in countries where people consumed more salt. In 1996, the same data was reviewed again. Researchers concluded that the link between blood pressure and salt was even stronger than first noted, especially in middle-aged and older people. Eating less salt, researchers said, could substantially reduce rates of heart disease.

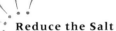

Clear the Confusion
Although the words salt and sodium are often used interchangeably, they are not the same. Salt, or more specifically table salt, is made up of about 60% chloride and 40% sodium. It is just one source of sodium in the diet.

Reduce the Salt
If you have thrown out the salt shaker in hopes of significantly reducing your salt intake, that's great, but it may not be enough. The majority of salt (as much as 75%) in most people's diets comes from processed and prepackaged foods, while about 10% occurs naturally in food. Only about 15% comes from the salt shaker.

The "I'm Not Salt-Sensitive" Controversy

In contrast to the conclusions of the Intersalt study, researchers from the University of Toronto recently analyzed 56 studies taken over 20 years and concluded that while it makes sense for people with high blood pressure to reduce their salt intake, there is no need for healthy people (those with normal blood pressure) to curtail their salt use. What's the best advice? The majority of health experts recommend moderate use of salt for several reasons. First, there are absolutely no health benefits to a diet high in salt. Second, even when you look beyond high blood pressure, research suggests that excess salt may increase the risk of diseases such as osteoporosis. Third, the only time you can tell whether excess salt will cause your blood pressure to rise is after you develop high blood pressure. In other words, why take the chance today, only to develop high blood pressure tomorrow?

Bottom line: At this time, around the world, there is a consensus that modest salt restriction is good for overall health and well-being.

> **News Flash: Potassium Update** Eating too much salt and too little potassium increases your chances of high blood pressure. The best way to increase your potassium intake is to max out in the fruit and vegetable category. Some great sources of potassium include dried apricots, prunes, potatoes, sweet potatoes, squash, orange juice – and of course, good old bananas.

How Much Salt?

For optimal health, most people should limit their sodium intake to about 2,400 mg per day, the amount found in about 1 teaspoon of salt. Most Canadians consume almost twice that amount. To reduce your intake, use the following foods in moderation: canned goods, snack foods, frozen dinners, soups, pickles, condiments, crackers, cheese, cold cuts and fast foods. Don't be reluctant to buy reduced-salt ver-

Reduce the Salt
Don't expect your tongue to tell you how much salt there is in the foods you eat. Many foods loaded with salt don't taste salty at all. Most frozen dinners, for example, score high on the salt index, yet one might not think so by taste alone. The best advice: when shopping, check labels and compare brands to help lower the amount of salt you use.

Reduce the Salt
Who says less salty means less tasty? Be creative and experiment with different herbs, spices and other flavour enhancers, like garlic and onions. Certain flavours substitute for salt better than others. Sour flavours, for instance, can replace a salty flavour. That's why lemon juice and vinegar are considered acceptable alternatives to salt. My sister rarely uses a salt shaker, but quite happily squirts lemon juice on just about every food in sight. Here's to happy squirting!

Read the Label

If you are reading an ingredient list, don't expect the word "salt" to represent the amount of sodium in a product. Quite often the sodium found in processed foods is in the form of ingredients such as sodium bicarbonate, monosodium phosphate, monosodium glutamate, and others.

Reduce the Salt

When choosing a salt substitute, pick the herbal blends rather than the potassium-based salt substitutes. Most of the potassium containing substitutes taste bitter instead of salty and just make you miss salt more. Better still, give yourself time to get used to a lower-salt diet. After a few weeks, you'll find the taste of most salty foods is, well, just too salty.

sions of your favourite products whenever possible. Studies have shown that salt can be reduced by 30 to 50% without affecting taste and consumer acceptability. And remember, if it's prepackaged and processed, it's also high in salt.

Salt Land Mines

Reminder – limit your daily sodium intake to about 2,400 mg per day.

	Sodium (mg)
Sauerkraut, canned (1 cup)	1560
Tomato sauce, canned (1 cup)	1480
Ham and Swiss sandwich (5 oz)	1350
Spaghetti sauce, bottled (1 cup)	1200
Potatoes au gratin (1 cup)	1065
Anchovies, canned (1 oz)	1050
Soy sauce (1 tbsp)	1030
Pinto beans, canned (1 cup)	1000
Turkey pot pie, frozen (8 oz)	1000
Macaroni and cheese, frozen (8 oz)	970
Green olives, small (10)	935
Cottage cheese (1 cup)	920
Chicken sandwich, fast-food	900
Big Mac or Whopper	880
Vegetable juice cocktail (1 cup)	880
Chicken soup, canned (1 cup)	870
Dill pickle (2 oz)	835
Baking soda (1 tsp)	820
Smoked sausage (2 oz)	800
Smoked herring (3 oz)	800
Imitation crabmeat (3 oz)	715
Canadian bacon (1.5 oz)	700
Gravy, canned (1/2 cup)	675

Source: University of California at Berkeley Wellness Letter, November 1996

What If I Don't Get Enough

With all this talk about too much salt in the diet, it's important to remember that sodium plays an important role in the control of fluid balance, nerve function and even muscle movement. If you're worried about not getting enough, however, put all your concerns aside. The minimum daily requirement for sodium for most adults is less than 100 mg, an easy amount to obtain since small amounts of sodium are naturally present in such a wide variety of foods.

In a Nutshell...

For optimal health, including a lower risk of high blood pressure, use salt in moderation. The majority of salt in the Canadian diet comes from processed and prepackaged foods.

Read the Label
A claim that a product contains less salt means the product is lower in salt but not necessarily low in salt. For example, "lite" soya sauce contains about 30% less salt than regular soya sauce. Although the "lite" brand is a better choice, it's still high in salt and should still be used in moderation.

Fifteen

Slim, Trim and Healthy

Top Twelve Things You Should Know about Weight Loss

1. Don't Blame It on Genetics

While genetics can influence how easily you gain weight, it does not destine anyone to a lifetime of fatness. How much weight individuals gain is still determined very much by what they eat and their level of activity. As an example, the Arizona Pima Indians and the Mexican Pima Indians share the same genetic makeup. And yet 75% of the Arizona Pima Indians suffer from obesity, while the average Mexican Pima Indian weighs 50 pounds less. Why the difference? The high-fat diet and inactive lifestyle of the Arizona Indians supports the accumulation of body fat. In contrast, the Mexican Pima Indians consume a low-fat diet and are active most of the time.

"Most of us don't know what poor losers we are until we try dieting."
Thomas Lamance

Clear the Confusion
Moderation doesn't mean giving up foods you enjoy, it only means having a smaller amount less often. It's not just what you eat, but how often and how much, that really makes the difference.

News Flash: Excess Body Fat Around the world, waistlines continue to expand at an alarming rate. In the last 10 years alone North Americans have gained an average of nearly 8 pounds per person. Approximately one third of Canadians are now obese. Even scarier is the fact that health professionals expect these numbers to continue to increase.

Weight Loss Tip
Strength training, such as lifting weights, helps to build and maintain muscle mass. The more muscle mass you have, the more calories you burn, even at rest.

2. Live Longer, Lose Weight

Slogans such as "I love my body – every gorgeous inch of it" can be found on everything from T-shirts to coffee mugs. Although our society does need to get away from the view that fat is bad, thin is good and blondes have more fun, we also have to recognize the overwhelming evidence that excess body weight negatively affects health and longevity. Overweight people are at much greater risk of developing chronic diseases such as heart disease and diabetes, as well as physical liabilities such as osteoarthritis. The good news is that even moderate weight loss can make a difference.

3. Is Your Weight Healthy?

What is a healthy weight? It's a weight that's right for the shape you were born with (your body build). It's a weight that's neither too fat nor too thin. It's a weight at which you feel healthy and energetic. And it's a weight at which you reduce your risk of disease. To determine if your weight is healthy, use the "Rate Your Weight" chart (p.127) to figure out your Body Mass Index (BMI). Simply select your height (in feet/inches across the bottom, or centimetres across the top) and follow its vertical line until it crosses the horizontal line of your body weight (pounds on the left side, kilograms on the right).

News Flash: Healthy Weight Are you an apple or a pear? It's better to be pear-shaped (bigger around the hips and thighs than the waist) than apple-shaped (bigger around the waist than the hips). Excess upper body weight is linked to a greater risk of heart disease, diabetes, high blood pressure and possibly some cancers.

How to interpret your BMI

BMI of less than 20   This is the underweight zone. You may not be getting enough calories and nutrients to meet your needs for good health. In addition, if changes in your weight are due to lack of appetite, a visit to your family physician is recommended in order to rule out any underlying problems.

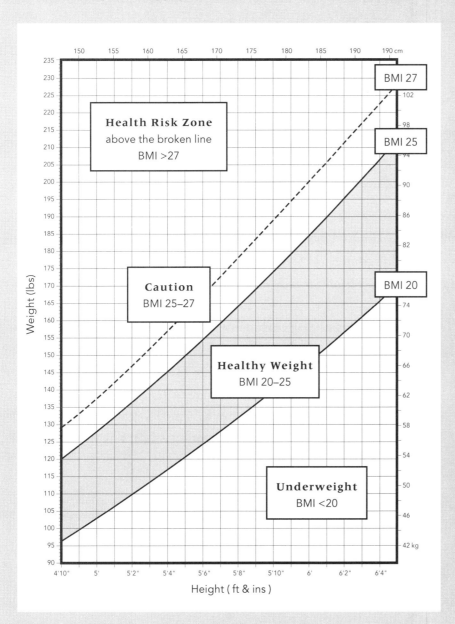

BMI between 20 and 25 This is the healthy weight zone. Give yourself a pat on the back. You are at low risk for health problems.

BMI between 25 and 27 This is the caution zone. Further weight gain is not recommended. You are at moderate risk for health problems.

BMI greater than 27 This is the high-risk zone. You should consider losing some weight. You are at high risk for health problems such as heart disease, high blood pressure and diabetes. The higher your BMI goes above 27, the greater your risk.

Please note: This chart is meant to be used by adults 20 to 65 years of age. Its should not be used with children, teens, pregnant or breastfeeding women, seniors, very muscular people or endurance athletes.

Source: Nutrition Services, Ottawa-Carleton Health Department, 1987. Revised 1994.

4. Healthy Weight Loss Equals Healthy Eating

Healthy weight loss is about enjoying food and accepting that your body deserves to be fed. It's about feeling satisfied at the end of a meal and taking delight in your favourite foods. It does not mean going hungry, skipping meals or binge-eating. Elaborate meal plans telling you to what to eat and when to eat it are not required. Liquid meals, diet pills and special food combinations are unnecessary. What is required? A diet that is low in fat, well balanced, and rich in fruits, vegetables and whole grains. Doesn't that sound like a diet you can live with?

5. Calories Still Count

Although reducing the amount of fat in your diet is important, many people mistakenly equate low-fat foods with a licence to eat. In a study from Penn State University, women were given a container of yogurt 30 minutes before lunch. When the women ate the yogurts labelled "low-fat," they consumed significantly more calories during the subsequent lunch and dinner than they did after eating the yogurt labelled "high fat." When the yogurts weren't labelled for fat content, these differences did not occur. These results are not surprising. People often eat low-fat foods, pat themselves on the back and feel they can indulge. Others think, "If it's low-fat, I can eat as much as I want." The truth is, low-fat foods can help promote weight loss, but only if eaten in reasonable amounts.

> **News Flash: The Milkshake Study** As part of a controlled study, 40 dieters and 40 nondieters were given 2 milkshakes to drink followed by an offer of ice cream. The dieters finished their milkshakes and ate the ice cream too. The nondieters ate very little ice cream once they finished the milkshakes. Why the difference? Nondieters tend to be much more in tune with their natural appetites, while chronic dieters tend to ignore or distrust inner signals of hunger or fullness.

6. Dieting Results in the "Last Supper" Mentality

It's Sunday evening, you have decided that tomorrow, Monday morning, once and for all, you are going to start your diet. So what do you do? You pig out. You gorge yourself on all your favourite foods. You eat well past the point of being full. You eat ice cream. You eat chocolate. You eat an entire bag of cookies. And then comes Monday morning. One of your co-workers walks in with a box of fresh doughnuts. How can you resist? You decide that perhaps you should start your diet on Tuesday, which means that today you had better enjoy all those fattening, forbidden foods that you soon will be unable to eat. The funny thing is, at the end of the week, you've actually eaten more food than you would have had you decided that dieting wasn't for you.

> **News Flash: Overweight Children** An overweight child is much more likely to become an overweight adult. It has been estimated that 40% of children who are overweight at age 7 become overweight adults, while 70 to 80% of overweight adolescents continue to be overweight as adults.

A good meal ought to begin with hunger.

7. Eat When You're Hungry (What a Concept!)

Pretend you are a car and your stomach is a gas tank: zero is empty, no fuel, nothing to go on. Ten is so full you can't put any more fuel into the tank. Five is half full. Now rate your hunger at this moment. Try this same test over the next several days. Tune in before, during and after each meal. Then answer this question: are you eating mostly when you're hungry? Or are you eating because you're bored, stressed, tired, depressed or lonely? Don't be an emotional eater.

8. Fill 'Er Up

Studies confirm that an expanding waistline is often linked to a low fibre intake (and vice versa). Most recently, researchers from the University of Sydney in Australia devised a Satiety Index based on how full volunteers felt after eating 240 calories' worth of various foods. Calorie for calorie, bulky, high-fibre foods such as fruits and vegetables rated high (people felt full longer after eating them). High-fat foods, on the other hand, tended to rank very low. Here are some of the findings:

Potatoes came out as the most filling food.

Whole grain bread was found to be twice as filling as white bread.

Cakes, doughnuts, croissants, candy bars, potato chips and ice cream all received poor marks for hunger satisfaction.

Fruit received high marks, with apples and oranges topping the list.

Popcorn received the best score in the snack category for filling you up.

> **News Flash: Reduce Your Waistline** A bowl of soup before your meal may help tip the scales in your favour. Research suggests that soup has the ability to turn off the appetite with far fewer calories than many other foods.

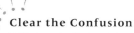

Clear the Confusion
Will chronic dieting (also referred to as yo-yo dieting) make you fat? Past diets do not seem to make it harder to lose weight or to make regaining it more rapid. Concerns about the hazards of weight cycling shouldn't deter anyone from trying to control their body weight.

9. Slow and Steady Wins the Race

"Lose 10 Pounds in Ten Days." "Drop 5 Pounds While You Sleep." "Lose-a-Pound-a-Day Diet." If you come across a headline that promises tremendous weight loss in a short period of time, do yourself a favour: ignore it. Studies show that small, consistent changes in both your eating habits and your level of activity are the best and most enjoyable route to long-term weight loss success. Healthy weight loss involves 1 to 2 kilograms (2–4 pounds) or less per week.

10. The Best Offence Is a Good Defence

If you have one potato chip, do you have to eat the whole bag? Is there a certain time of the day when you tend to get so hungry you'll eat anything in sight? If you know when you're most likely to overindulge, you can avoid it. For example, if one chip leads to a bag, perhaps you should avoid chips altogether. If you're always hungry in late afternoon, keep a supply of healthy snacks on hand to curb the urge to splurge. In other words, identify your areas of weakness and then develop a plan that makes winning easy.

> **News Flash: Unrealistic Body Image**   Some of the models seen on the covers of women's magazines have described their food intake the week prior to a camera shoot as "a cracker for lunch, a cracker for dinner, and maybe a few boiled vegetables." How healthy does that sound?

11. It's Okay to Indulge

For the next 5 minutes, keep your left leg perfectly still. Don't move it even 1 inch. What happens at the end of 5 minutes? You move your leg. In fact, after being told *not* to move it, keeping it still becomes almost unbearable. Let's translate this into the world of food. Let's assume that I told you that you could never eat chocolate again. Guess what happens? You think about chocolate. You dream about chocolate. You have cravings for chocolate. And when you actually get your hands on some of the stuff you devour it with wild abandon. Now let's look at an alternative scenario. Let's say that I tell you chocolate is perfectly acceptable. I even let you know that I understand your love of chocolate and I appreciate your need for what you call your regular "chocolate fix." My only request is that you go easy on the quantities of chocolate consumed. In addition, I provide you with some low-fat, chocolate-like alternatives, like Tootsie Rolls, that can be substituted for chocolate at least some of the time. Sound better? We shouldn't feel guilty about the good stuff. Consumed in moderation, all foods have their place.

Clear the Confusion

Many people mistakenly believe that lower-intensity workouts (like walking) are better for burning body fat. Allow me to clarify. During prolonged low-intensity workouts a higher proportion of the calories burned come from fat (about 50%) as compared to higher intensity workouts (about 40%). However, since you burn many more calories during intense exercise, you ultimately end up burning more fat.

Bottom line: the longer and harder you work out, the more calories (and fat) you'll burn.

> **News Flash: Turn Off the Tube** In both adults and children excess television viewing equals excess weight. In one study women who watched 3 hours per day of television or more were twice as likely to be overweight than those who watched 1 hour per day or less. Another study found that the strongest predictor of weight regain following weight loss was frequent television viewing. Not only do we watch TV instead of doing something more active, TV creates a state of semi-consciousness that lowers the rate at which the body burns energy.

12. You've Got to Move

In this age of technological advancements – computers, portable telephones, garage door openers, televisions, remote controls, cars – activities of daily living have been severely reduced. As a result, our bodies burn far fewer calories than in the past, and our ability to maintain a healthy body weight is much more difficult. The solution? We need to make a conscious effort to move our bodies in an environment that provides little opportunity to do so. Regular physical activity is absolutely essential for weight maintenance, weight loss and good health.

> **News Flash: Weight Loss and Exercise** In a recent study from the University of Melbourne in Australia, people who exercised to lose weight lost a greater percentage of their weight as body fat (more than 80% of weight lost was body fat, less than 20% was lean body tissue) as compared to people who used diet alone (60% of weight lost was body fat, 40% was lean tissue).

> **News Flash: Prevent Weight Gain** Some researchers believe the best way to prevent weight gain is to make sure people are particularly careful not to gain weight during those periods in the life cycle when weight gain is most likely to occur. Adolescence, pregnancy, and menopause have been identified as three such times. With pregnancy, this refers to the weight gained above and beyond what is recommended for a healthy pregnancy – most women should gain 11 to 16 kilograms (25–35 pounds).

Don't Do It Alone

Oprah Winfrey made headlines with her weight loss. How did she do it? She had a personal chef who cooked up delicious low-fat meals, and she had a personal fitness trainer who worked out with her every morning and every afternoon. Although you probably can't afford such luxuries, it doesn't mean you have to go it alone. Here are some ways to get support:

See a Dietitian. A dietitian can provide a good primer course on how and what to eat, and design a program that suits your food preferences and lifestyle. A dietitian can also point out what changes in your diet will give you the biggest bang for your buck.

Join a Reputable Weight Loss Group Such as Weight Watchers. These groups provide not only a learning environment but also a strong support network for your weight loss efforts. Ideally, the program should be based on foods you cook and prepare yourself, not on prepackaged foods. It should be based on a balanced menu plan with a strong emphasis on regular physical activity. And, of course, it should have a strong emphasis not only on getting the weight off, but also on keeping it off.

Do It with a Buddy. Get a neighbour, friend or your spouse to join you in making changes in your lifestyle. Share tips and celebrate victories. Buddies make life more fun.

Top Ten Ways to Make Active Living a Part of Your Life

1. Think of the Benefits

Instead of focusing on why you can't or don't want to exercise, think about the benefits. Remember how great you feel at the end of a workout. Think about how much easier it is to control your weight. Focus on how much more energy you have, how much better you sleep at night, and how significantly you reduce your risk of heart disease, diabetes, osteoporosis and cancer.

"If exercise were a drug, it would be the most prescribed medicine in the world."

The National Institute of Aging

> **News Flash: Couch Potatoes Listen Up**   Research shows that people who derive the greatest benefits from physical activity are those who go from being completely inactive (true couch potatoes) to being moderately active. There has never been a better time to get off the couch and get moving.

2. Have Fun

Don't worry if it's high-impact, low-impact, butt-slimming or fat-burning. Find an activity you enjoy and do it on a regular basis. Personally, I love walking, I think step classes are fun and I could dance all night.

> **News Flash: Number of Overweight Children Increasing**
> As the waistline of the average Canadian expands, so does the waistline of the average Canadian child. The number of overweight children aged 6 to 11 has increased by an astounding 50% in the last 15 years. Not only are more youngsters overweight, they are more severely overweight than ever before. Research strongly suggests that the increasing rates of obesity in our children has more to do with a decrease in their physical activity than with an increase in their food intake.

3. Start Slow

Don't jump in the deep end or try to jog 5 kilometres the first day. If your initial attempt at physical activity is too aggressive, you are much more likely to get discouraged and drop out (not to mention the fact that you'll find it painful to walk for the next week).

> **News Flash: Unrealistic Body Image**   Many of the stars we see in the movies with what some would call the "perfect body" spend 2 to 5 hours exercising each day.

4. Think Regular

Think of physical activity in the same way you would think about having a shower. Most people shower daily, and rarely skip a day. Your approach to active living should be the same. It's not how *hard* you work out, but how *regularly,* that most benefits your health.

5. Get Social

When you work out with a buddy, you are much more likely to start an exercise program in the first place and far more likely to stick with it down the road. For pleasure and inspiration, exercise with friends.

6. Mix It Up

Just as eating the same foods every day can get pretty boring, so can the same exercise routine. Don't do the same thing every day. Go walking, jogging, hiking, biking. Change your music, change your walking route, change your running shoes.

7. Have an Indoor Alternative

In Canada, winter is cold with a capital "C." Have an indoor alternative. Join a fitness club. Get a treadmill. Go mall walking.

8. Make a Date with a Personal Fitness Trainer

A certified fitness trainer can design a program that suits your needs and your lifestyle. He or she can show you how to exercise efficiently, properly and safely. And a fitness trainer can give you that extra little push to get you started.

Goal Setting Tip
I'm a big believer in setting goals. However, goals that say "I will never eat chocolate again" or "I will exercise every single day of the entire year" encourage "all or nothing" behaviour. If you have a piece of chocolate or if you miss one day of exercising, you feel like a failure and are tempted to throw in the towel. Bottom line: set realistic goals with realistic time frames that allow for the occasional slip.

Bonus Tip – Man's Best Friend
A University of Guelph study of more than 1,000 people found that pet owners are more active, fitter and healthier than non-pet owners. Perhaps it's time for man's best friend and walking partner – time to get a dog.

9. Sweat In Tune

An Ohio State University study found that people exercise 25 to 30% longer when they listen to music. Music makes you want to move. It makes exercise more fun. Whether you like Frank Sinatra, Elvis Presley, Blue Rodeo or Alvin and the Chipmunks, turn on the music, sing along and sweat in tune.

10. It All Counts

You've heard it before: take the stairs instead of the elevator, leave your car at the far end of the parking lot. The truth is you don't have to be an Olympic athlete to experience the incredible benefits of active living. In fact, physical activity need not be vigorous to improve health. Current guidelines recommend that people of all ages include a minimum of 30 minutes of physical activity of moderate intensity (a brisk walk versus a slow stroll) on most, if not all, days of the week. These 30 minutes don't have to be all at the same time – 10 minutes here, 10 minutes there, it all adds up – it all counts.

In a Nutshell...

Excess body weight is a growing problem for both adults and children. The best way to achieve a healthy body weight is through healthy eating and active living. A healthy diet is low in fat, well balanced, and abundant in fruits, vegetables and whole grains. Healthy eating means eating when you're hungry, stopping when you're full. Active living means participating in activities you enjoy on a regular basis.

Sixteen

The Pill-Popping Question

Top Four Reasons to Approach Supplements with Caution

About 4 out of every 10 Canadians take vitamin or mineral supplements on a regular basis. If you are one of them, here are four things to consider when evaluating your pill-popping habits.

1. Pill Popping Can Upset Nature's Natural Balance

Vitamins and minerals should be handled with care. Nature has packaged the perfect dosage and combination of vitamins and minerals in food. Pill popping can upset this delicate balance, especially if you take large doses of individual nutrients. For example, too much zinc interferes with the absorption of both copper and iron. And too much beta-carotene can affect blood levels of lycopene (another carotenoid that's important to optimal health).

"Let food be your medicine and medicine be your food."
Hippocrates, 400 B.C.

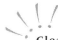

2. Pill Popping Can Be Dangerous

The phrase "a little is good, so more must be better" doesn't apply to pill popping. In large doses, the dangers of toxicity can outweigh the possibility of any so-called miracle effects. This is especially true when it comes to vitamin A, vitamin D, vitamin B6, iron, zinc and selenium. Even at relatively low doses, vitamin A during pregnancy can cause birth defects. Large doses of vitamin B6 can lead to partial paralysis. High-dose niacin supplements can cause liver damage. And the list goes on.

3. A Pill and Food Are Not the Same

A pill does not provide the same benefits as food. For example, studies have shown that a diet rich in beta-carotene-containing foods, like fruits and vegetables, significantly reduces the risk of both heart disease and cancer. Because of this research, a large study involving 29,000 male smokers was undertaken in Finland to look at the benefits of beta-carotene in a supplement form. The results were both shocking and disappointing. After 5 to 8 years, the beta-carotene takers had an 18% higher risk of lung cancer. Subsequent studies showed similar disappointing results. Because of these results, organizations such as the Center for Science in the Public Interest, which had previously recommended beta-carotene supplements, changed their point of view. While studies related to vitamin E have been more promising, further long-term research is required before a vitamin or mineral in a pill form can be recommended for the prevention of disease or for optimal health.

News Flash: Vitamin C and the Common Cold Based on a review of 20 studies, it appears that while vitamin C will not prevent colds, it can lessen the severity and duration of cold symptoms.

4. Good Nutrition Can't Be Bottled

The science of nutrition is still in its infancy. Every day, researchers discover new compounds, like phytochemicals, that may play an essential role in optimal health. *Newsweek* said it best: "Whole natural foods harbor a whole ratatouille of compounds that have never seen the inside of a vitamin bottle for the simple reason that scientists have not, until very recently, even known they existed, let alone brewed them into pills." In other words, if you are looking for the most powerful combination of vitamins, minerals, antioxidants, fibre and phytochemicals, the best place to find them is in food.

> **News Flash: Red Alert! Keep Vitamin Pills out of Reach**
> Vitamin pills containing iron are the leading cause of poisoning deaths in small children. Keep your vitamin pills out of sight and out of reach.

Clear the Confusion
Experts say there's no convincing evidence that the supplements that contain minerals in "chelated" or "colloidal" form are better absorbed or utilized by the body.

Six Reasons to Consider a Vitamin or Mineral Supplement

Most people can get the vitamins and minerals they need from eating a well-balanced diet that includes milk products, whole grains, fruits and vegetables, and meat and alternatives. Here are six situations where a vitamin or mineral supplement may be required.

1. *Vitamin B12* (2 mcg/day) should be taken by strict vegetarians who don't eat any animal products.
2. *Vitamin D* (100–400 I.U./day) should be taken by those with limited milk intake and sunlight exposure.
3. *Calcium* (500–1,000 mg/day) should be taken by those with milk allergies and may be required by those who suffer from lactose intolerance. Further research will tell us whether individuals at high risk for osteoporosis, such as postmenopausal women, may benefit from a calcium supplement.

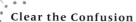

Super Nutrition Tip
Most vitamin pills should be taken with meals, rather than on an empty stomach, for maximum nutrient absorption.

4. *Folic acid* (.4 mg/day) should be taken by women planning to get pregnant if their diet is not rich in grains (breads, cereals, pasta), beans and leafy greens. For greatest benefit, begin one month before conception and continue through the first trimester. Folic acid helps to prevent certain birth defects, called neural tube defects, that affect the brain and spinal cord.

5. *Iron and calcium* from a prenatal supplement may benefit pregnant women.

6. *In terms of antioxidants, vitamin E* (100–400 I.U./day) may be beneficial for those who are at high risk for heart disease, although further research in this area is required. Most nutrition experts recommend that needs for both beta-carotene and vitamin C be met through a diet rich in fruits and vegetables.

It is always a good idea to consult with a dietitian to determine whether a supplement is required and what the appropriate dosage is.

Clear the Confusion
There is nothing magical about meal replacement drinks (liquid nutritional supplements). Most are simply skim milk, water, sugars, vegetable oil, thickeners and flavouring agents, plus some vitamins and minerals. They may be healthier than a candy bar or a bag of chips, but a container of yogurt and a piece of fruit can be just as easy and convenient when you're on the run or filling in the gaps.

Should You Take a Multi-Vitamin?

With the exception of the University of California at Berkeley, which recommends that all adults take supplements for vitamin E (200–800 I.U.) and vitamin C (250–500 mg), no other scientific body of nutrition experts, including the Dietitians of Canada and the American Dietetic Association, recommends that everyone take supplements on a routine basis as dietary insurance or for optimal health. If, however, you choose to use supplements, most nutrition experts suggest you do so at levels that do not exceed your recommended daily requirement. Overall, the best way to do this is with a multi-vitamin. The average multi-vitamin supplement contains relatively safe amounts of a wide variety of nutrients.

In a Nutshell...

Eating food is the best way to optimize health, prevent disease and meet nutritional requirements. There are certain times when a vitamin or mineral supplement is warranted. More research is required before vitamin and mineral supplements can be recommended for disease prevention.

Seventeen

Life in the Fast Lane

Top Ten Convenience Foods

For those days when you don't have time to cook, here are some simple ideas for putting good food on the table fast. Do, however, keep in mind that most convenience foods should be consumed in moderation, since most are high in salt.

1. Salad-in-a-Bag

If you buy your salads already washed, cut and bagged, don't feel guilty. These salads are both nutritious and convenient. Most of the plastic wraps and bags used for packaging these products are specially engineered to maximize nutrient retention and keep the produce fresh. Veggies and dip are another easy option. Simply use bagged, peeled baby carrots and a low-fat salad dressing for dipping.

"Life is too short to stuff a mushroom."

Shirley Conran

Shopping Trivia
The "average" main grocery trip takes place in the afternoon towards the end of the week, lasts about 45 minutes and consists of about 30 items.

Super Nutrition Tip
What is a balanced meal anyway?
Try to eat at least 3 of the 4 food
groups – milk products, grains, fruits
and vegetables, and meat or meat
alternatives – at every meal. It's easier
than it sounds. For example, rather
than having just eggs for dinner,
round out the meal with a couple of
pieces of whole wheat toast and a
glass of milk. Finish it off with a piece
of fruit.

Time Tip
Put cooking time to good use by
making a big batch of brown rice and
freezing some of it. Cooked rice
stores up to 7 days in the fridge and 6
months in the freezer. To reheat, add
2 tablespoons (30 mL) water per cup
cooked rice; microwave (thawed) rice
and liquid about 1½ minutes or heat
on stove top 4 to 5 minutes.

Shopping Trivia
By and large, women make the
decisions about what we eat at
home. Eighty-five per cent of women
do the grocery shopping. About the
same number do the cooking at
dinnertime.

2. More Beans, Please

Here are five fast and easy ways to eat more beans:

1. Why make plain rice, when it's just as easy to make beans and rice? Both Uncle Ben's and President's Choice have a complete line of beans and rice side dishes. Just add water and heat.

2. President's Choice One Step Pasta and Beans is as easy to prepare as Kraft Dinner and can serve as either a side dish or a main meal.

3. Simply heat up a can of baked beans in tomato sauce. It doesn't get any easier than that.

4. Ready-made bean dips (such as hummus) are widely available. Serve them with whole wheat pita bread.

5. Canned, ready-to-serve, marinated bean salads, such as Insalata Toscana by Unico, are simply delicious.

3. Be a Fish Eater

Here are four fast and easy ways to eat more fish:

1. Fresh or frozen fish fillets, from cod to sole to bluefish to salmon, are widely available. Try the recipe on p.195 with your favourite fish for a particularly quick and tasty meal.

2. If it's breaded fish you're looking for, try Healthy Bake by High Liner. It's available in both fish sticks and fish fillets. Unlike most breaded fish, it's baked, not deep-fried.

3. Both fresh and frozen fish fillets can be purchased already seasoned. BlueWater Seafoods, for example, has frozen Grilled Fish Fillets that come in flavours like lemon herb, lemon pepper and Italian herb.

4. Ready-made salmon burgers can be grilled on the barbecue in no time.

4. Stir-Fries Made Easy

Making a stir-fry has never been so easy. Simply use frozen vegetables and boneless chicken breasts (thawed) and a low-fat stir-fry sauce such as Uncle Ben's Sweet & Sour or Teriyaki. It's as easy as one, two, three.

> **News Flash: Smart Refrigerators**   *Food Processing* magazine predicts that someday soon your refrigerator will not only store food, it will choose it and restrict it, too. Computerized "smart" refrigerators, programmed with personal codes, will withhold goodies and snacks if they don't think we should have them. Doesn't sound like much fun to me.

5. Pizza, Anyone?

What would you say to pizza that's lower in fat than your typical take-out or frozen pizza and also ready in minutes? Simply use a ready-made flatbread, such as President's Choice Thindido or Master Choice Crustino as the crust. Cover lightly with any canned or bottled tomato sauce. Sprinkle lightly with partly-skimmed Mozzarella cheese (look for "15% M.F." on the label and buy the pre-grated kind). Add whatever toppings you like and pop in the oven for less than 10 minutes.

6. Frozen Dinners

Most supermarkets offer a wide selection of individual frozen dinners. Although it's almost impossible to get away from the high salt content of these meals, you can stick to those brands that are lower in fat, such as Weight Watchers Healthy Gourmet, Weight Watchers Smart Ones, Stouffer's Lean Cuisine and President's Choice Too Good To Be True. In terms of lower-fat, family-size frozen dinners, the selection here is poor. Once again, President's Choice is the leader with products such as Too Good To Be True Ratatouille, Paella, Pad Thai and Jambalaya.

Time Tip
Ten super-fast meals: cereal, soup, eggs, pancakes, French toast, a sandwich, pasta with ready-made sauce, a frozen dinner, fish, and boneless chicken breasts on the barbecue.

Time Tip
Potatoes baked in the microwave are fast and easy. Simply prick the skin and cook on high for 3 to 4 minutes for 1 potato. After microwaving, wrap in a tea towel for 5 to 10 minutes while you prepare the rest of the meal. For crispier skin, place the cooked potatoes in the oven for about 10 minutes. Salsa, low-fat tzatziki and low-fat sour cream make great potato toppings.

Super Nutrition Tip
Don't always wait until the last minute to decide what to eat. People who plan their meals ahead of time find it easier to eat a balanced, healthy diet, and feel better about their overall health.

Schneiders also has some entries with their Stir-Fry and Fajita Kits. Let your family be the judge.

7. Spaghetti and Sauce

Boil the spaghetti, heat the sauce, add a sprinkle of Parmesan and you're there. Just a few points to consider: First, choose whole wheat pasta like Catelli Healthy Harvest Whole Wheat Spaghetti. Second, look for those tomato sauces that are both low in fat (most of them are) and lower in salt (hard to find). Good examples include Healthy Choice pasta sauces and President's Choice Too Good To Be True sauces. Most premixed pasta and sauce meals are too high in fat.

8. Soup's On

A bowl of soup makes a quick meal that can be both hearty and nutritious, especially when it's rich in both vegetables and beans. Minestrone is the perfect example. Serve it alongside whole wheat bread and a glass of milk. My personal favourite is Minestrone Soupworks by Lipton. It's both low in fat and delicious. Just a reminder – almost all store-bought soups are high in salt.

9. Chicken Fingers in a Flash

Cut boneless chicken breasts into strips or cubes, roll them in a coating mix such as Shake 'n' Bake, and pop them in the oven. You've got low-fat chicken fingers or nuggets in 15 minutes or less. A honey mustard or plum sauce can be used for dipping.

10. Macaroni and Cheese in a Box – A Lighter Version of a Family Favourite

Kids love it. Moms love it. Dads love it. A lot of people love the taste and convenience of macaroni and cheese, also known as Kraft Dinner.

What's more, by making a few minor modifications in its preparation, this family favourite can be lightened up substantially. It's really quite simple. When mixing the cheese sauce, rather than adding the 3 tablespoons (45 mL) of butter or margarine called for in the directions, add only 2 teaspoons (10 mL) and a touch more milk. This small change will reduce the fat content of each $^3/_4$ cup serving from 11 grams of fat to about 4 grams of fat (that's a difference of 7 fat grams per serving!). Apply this logic whenever possible when following package directions.

In a Nutshell...

There are many convenience foods now available that allow you to make quick, nutritious meals in minutes. Because of their high salt content, use them in moderation.

Ten Commandments of Dining Out

1. Before You Go

The first step to healthy eating on the town takes place before you step out the door. It involves choosing a restaurant that offers healthy food options. If you're out of town, or unfamiliar with the restaurants in your area, don't feel shy about calling ahead to review the menu.

2. Watch Out for the "What the Heck" Syndrome

Many of us view dining out as a special treat, and therefore an excuse to overindulge. "What the heck," we say, "it's only one meal. I might as well go for it." We then proceed to order the large Caesar salad, followed by the fettuccine Alfredo, and a huge piece of double chocolate fudge cake for the grand finale. Over 2,000 calories and 150 grams of fat later, we undo the top button of our pants in order to relieve the

Dining Out Trivia
On average, Canadians eat out 4.75 times per week (this includes breakfast, lunch and dinner) which means restaurants serve approximately 135 million meals every week.

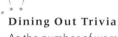

pressure. While I don't suggest you deny yourself all pleasures, a little restraint will avoid both clogged arteries and a bigger waistline later on. The occasional splurge is one thing, but if you eat out quite often, try to limit your intake most of the time. In the end, you can have your cake and eat it too (just not every day).

3. Become Menu Literate

Descriptions of foods on the menu can be misleading. Good words to look for include: *broiled, roasted, grilled, poached, steamed, charbroiled, marinara, primavera, tomato-based, marinated/cooked in juice, marinated/cooked in wine.*

Not-so-good words include: *fried, crispy, au gratin (with cheese), marinated/cooked in oil, marinated/cooked in butter, breaded, sautéed, pan-fried, butter sauce, cream sauce, Alfredo, hollandaise, béarnaise, dipped in batter, served in pastry.*

4. Assert Yourself

When you eat out, you are not at the mercy of the chef. Ask your waiter or waitress what the dishes contain if you are unsure, and order your food prepared and served the way you want it. Here are a few suggestions:

Request sauces and dressings be served on the side.
Request your food be prepared with little or no fat.
Request rice or a baked potato instead of French fries.
Request milk for your coffee instead of cream.
Ask for whole grains rolls or bread instead of white.
Ask for a side dish of vegetables if the entrée doesn't
   include them.

> **News Flash: Dining Out = Poor Nutrition**   Studies suggest
> that increased consumption of food away from home contributes to
> a higher intake of fat and calories and a reduced intake of fibre, cal-
> cium, vitamin C and folic acid.

5. Don't Eat It Just Because It's There

When asked why he wanted to climb Mount Everest, George Leigh
Mallory said, "Because it is there." Be very careful not to apply this
reasoning to restaurant meals. The portion sizes in most restaurants
are just too big. If you suffer from "clean plate syndrome," you'll probably consume twice the amount of food you actually need.
Fortunately, you have several options. Ask for an extra plate and share
the meal with a friend. Order one or two appetizers and skip the main
meal entirely. Request a doggie bag and then use it. Most important:
don't eat it just because it's there.

> **News Flash: Dining Out Mega Meals**   Generally speaking,
> meals eaten at restaurants are significantly larger and contain a
> higher proportion of fat than meals eaten at home.

6. Beware the Buffet Table

Most people tend to eat more food when it's served buffet style. With
so many foods to choose from and so many wonderful things to try, it's
almost impossible to avoid overindulgence. Your best bet is to
approach the buffet table as a visual menu, rather than an invitation to
try everything. However, if, like me, you feel compelled to taste a bit of
everything, make sure your portions are very small. Happy tasting.

7. Be an All-Star Eater

Dining well does not have to damage your arteries or your waistline.
Here are some basic guidelines for healthier, low-fat fare.

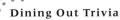

Dining Out Trivia
The top 10 food items ordered from restaurants and foodservice outlets are French fries, salad, pizza, baked goods, hamburgers, sweetened baked goods, sandwiches, dessert, ice cream, soup. (Canadian Restaurant and Foodservices Association, 1995.)

1. Choose clear soups, especially those loaded with veggies or beans.
2. Have a skinless turkey or chicken breast.
3. Enjoy a small filet mignon or sirloin steak.
4. Tomato-based sauces are a must on the pasta front.
5. Fajitas get top marks as long as you go easy on the guacamole and sour cream.
6. Veggie-loaded stir-fries offer great taste and nutrition.
7. As long as it's not breaded and fried, seafood gets top marks on the health front.
8. Approach all salads with caution. Order a light salad dressing "on the side."

8. More People Means More Food

Who you dine with and how many people are at the table can significantly increase how much food you eat. For example, research shows if you dine with someone who eats a large amount of food, you may increase your intake by as much as 25 to 69%. Therefore, when in the company of a big eater, be careful of the tendency to eat more than you normally would. It's also wise to watch your intake at large social gatherings. Studies indicate that as the number of people at the table increases, so does the average amount of food consumed. This is fine if you attend large social events on an occasional basis. If you have the pleasure of regularly eating with a crowd, however, be aware of the "people effect" and watch your intake accordingly.

9. When in Flight, Order Right

For people who travel a lot, dining out often includes eating on airplanes. Unfortunately, a typical airline meal often contains more than 1,000 calories, and some of the 5-course meals offered in business or first class contain as many as 4,000 calories. Luckily, there are other options. All airlines now offer low-fat or light meals that can be ordered in advance. You can reserve one of these special meals when you make your plane reservation. And don't forget to drink at least one glass of water or juice for every hour in the air, to offset the dehydrating effects of flying.

10. The Grand Finale...Dessert

If you see me in a restaurant eating tiramisu, don't be shocked. Tiramisu is my all-time favourite dessert. It is, however, decadently rich (don't even ask how many fat grams it contains). That's why I don't eat it very often and when I do, I usually split it with my husband and savour each and every bite. Most of the time, however, I satisfy my dessert cravings with light options like these:

1. Fresh fruit in season is always divine and often beautifully presented.
2. Low-fat frozen yogurt, sherbet or sorbets are refreshingly light.
3. Angel food cake is surprisingly low in fat and great tasting too.
4. Gourmet dessert coffees or cappuccinos (made with low-fat milk) are very enjoyable.
5. (Highly recommended.) Skip dessert and go for a walk (now there's an idea!).

By the way, if you decide to skip dessert, I suggest you say no immediately when asked. It's too easy to change your mind and give in to sweet temptations. Just reading a dessert list is enough to push most people over the edge.

In a Nutshell...

Pick a restaurant that offers healthy food options. Order the healthy foods. Watch the tendency to eat more than you need.

Top Ten Fast-Food Survival Tips

1. Welcome to Fat Gram City

Most fast-food restaurants are a haven for fat grams. If you are an occasional visitor, it's not a problem. If, however, you visit on a more regular basis, you are most likely consuming more fat and more calories than you need. Healthy food options do exist, but most items on your average fast-food menu should be approached with caution.

2. Have Some Salt with Your Salt

Fast food can not only cause you to surpass your fat gram quota for the day in the blink of an eye, it can also provide mega quantities of salt. Let's do a quick recap on sodium (salt). The average person should try to limit his or her daily intake to about 2,400 milligrams per day. Now take a look at the sodium content of some popular fast-food items:

	Sodium mg
KFC Chicken Wings (6)	1,230
Wendy's Taco Salad	1,188
McDonald's Big Mac	1,047
Swiss Chalet Chicken Pot Pie	951
Pizza Hut Super Supreme Pan Pizza (1 medium slice)	826

The majority of fast-food items make a significant contribution on the salt front and should be consumed in moderation.

News Flash: Fast-Food Windows Are Hot   Drive-though windows at fast-food restaurants are thriving across the country. In fact, more people than ever are eating their meals in their cars, often while driving. Hey, you, don't forget to watch the road.

Fast-Food Trivia
About 70% of all restaurant meals are purchased from fast-food or counter service restaurants.

KFC

	Grams of fat
Chicken Pot Pie	40.0
Hot Wings (6)	33.0
Extra Crispy Tasty Chicken (breast)	27.0
Kentucky Nuggets (6)	18.0
Original Recipe Chicken (breast)	15.0

3. Where's the Broccoli?

Where's the broccoli? Yes, you can order broccoli on your baked potato. However, at Wendy's it comes with a large load of cheese sauce and a whopping 13 grams of fat per serving. Most meals at your average fast-food outlet are lacking in one or more of the major food groups. Fruits and vegetables are one area of weakness. (Sorry, French fries don't count.) Even salads are made primarily with iceberg lettuce (the nutritional weakling of the lettuce family) and then loaded with high-fat dressing. And while milk is always an option, soft drinks are usually the beverage of choice.

4. Proceed with Caution: Double Trouble, Special Sauces and Deep-Fried Foods

Here are some fat-reducing guidelines:

1. Go easy on the special sauces. Most are made with mayonnaise and contain about 11 grams of fat per tablespoon (15 mL).
2. Double meat patties and double cheese equal double trouble. More specifically, most double-decker mega burgers contain three times as much fat as their regular counterparts.
3. Don't assume that fish or chicken are healthier choices. They are usually breaded and deep fried. For example, a small hamburger at McDonald's has half the fat of a Filet-O-Fish.

> **News Flash: Empty Calorie All-Star**   If it's "empty calories" you are looking for, look no further than a large Coca-Cola from McDonald's. Containing more than 20 teaspoons (100 mL) of sugar per serving and nothing in the way of vitamins or minerals, it takes first place as the sugar-only all-star.

**McDonald's –
Pizza, McNuggets, Fries
and Salads**

	Grams of fat
Large fries	24.0
Pepperoni Personal Pizza	23.0
Garden Salad w/house dressing	21.0
Chicken McNuggets (6 pieces)	14.0
Garden Salad w/vinaigrette dressing	1.0

**McDonald's –
Sandwiches and Burgers**

	Grams of fat
Arch Deluxe w/bacon	34.0
Big Mac	30.0
McChicken	29.0
Filet-O-Fish	19.0
Hamburger	8.9

Reduce the Fat
Don't be fooled by the Veggies and Dip available at Swiss Chalet. The dip contains 26 grams of fat per serving. Best advice: get the veggies, hold the dip.

5. Salads and Fat: The Sky's the Limit

Don't be fooled into thinking salads are a "light" choice. The Caesar salad at Swiss Chalet contains almost 40 grams of fat per serving. On the other hand, the Quarter Chicken White, with the skin removed, a baked potato, a roll, and the Chalet Sauce used for dipping (only 1 gram of fat per serving!), contains only 10 grams of fat. High-fat salads are standard fare at fast-food restaurants. Reduced-fat salad dressings are, however, available. Best advice: when it comes to salad, go light or go home.

6. Better Breakfasts

Your best bets on the fast-food breakfast circuit are English muffins, low-fat muffins, bagels and pancakes – as long as you go easy on the butter. Some places even offer cereal, a very healthy choice! An Egg McMuffin, while not low in fat, contains half the fat of a Sausage McMuffin. Watch out for croissants and Danishes. They're swimming in fat. And for a nice dose of vitamin C and folic acid, don't forget to enjoy some orange juice with your meal.

7. The Perils of Pizza

The two villains in the pizza hall of fame are the meat toppings and the cheese. However, if you choose ham, rather than fatty meats, like sausage, bacon or ground beef, you'll save yourself as much as 9 grams of fat per slice. And many pizza places will go easy on the cheese. All you have to do is ask. To get some added goodness from your pizza, load up on the veggie front. Last but not least, the thinner crust pizzas tend to contain less fat than the popular pan-type varieties.

Swiss Chalet

	Grams of fat
Full Back Ribs	52.0
Caesar salad entree	38.0
Fries	22.0
1/4 Chicken White (with skin)	22.0
1/4 Chicken White (skinless)	8.0

McDonald's – Breakfast

	Grams of fat
Sausage McMuffin w/egg	26.0
Egg McMuffin	12.0
Hot Cakes w/butter and syrup	10.0
Fat-Wise cranberry orange muffin	9.5
English muffin w/margarine	4.5

Pizza Hut

Based on 1 slice of medium pizza

	Grams of fat
Meat Lover's Pan Pizza	18.0
Super Supreme Pan Pizza	17.0
Cheese Pan Pizza	11.0
Veggie Lover's Pan Pizza	10.0
Veggie Lover's Thin 'n' Crispy Pizza	7.0

8. *Three Cheers for the Grilled Chicken Sandwich*

Hip hip hooray! Yes, you can have your cake and eat it too. The best advice I can give you at the fast-food counter is get the grilled chicken sandwich. Not the breaded and deep-fried chicken sandwich. Not the chicken nuggets. The grilled chicken sandwich. This type of sandwich is available at many (not all) fast-food outlets. From an overall fat perspective it's the healthiest option going. The second best option is, quite simply, a plain hamburger. And replace the fries with a baked potato if that option exists (just avoid loading it with cheese). And last but not least, enjoy a bowl of chili (available at Wendy's) and get the goodness of beans.

9. *The Dessert Menu*

Your best choice on the dessert menu is either ice milk (get the regular cone, not the waffle cone) found at places like McDonald's, or low-fat frozen yogurt found at places like Dairy Queen. These desserts are relatively low in fat and provide a healthy dose of nutrients such as bone-building calcium. They also make a great snack any time of day.

10. *There's Hope on the Horizon*

As bleak as things seem, changes are coming. Fast-food outlets are responding to the changing needs of customers, and offering a better selection of healthy foods. And new fast-food outlets are opening that cater to healthy hearts and waistlines. An outlet by the name of O-Tooz (currently only in Toronto and Vancouver) serves up delicious fruit shakes, lower-fat sandwich fare, veggies wrapped in whole wheat tortillas, and desserts that are both light and tasty. The future is looking bright.

Wendy's	
	Grams of fat
Taco salad	30.0
Baked potato w/cheese sauce	22.0
Grilled chicken sandwich	6.8
Small chili	6.6
Baked potato w/sour cream and chives	4.3

McDonald's – Dessert	
	Grams of fat
Baked raspberry pie	20.0
McDonaldland cookies (box)	9.8
Vanilla ice milk – waffle cone	7.8
Hot fudge sundae – ice milk	7.3
Vanilla ice milk – regular cone	4.6

Super Nutrition Tip

Four suggestions for your next visit to a salad bar. First, load up on the veggies, romaine lettuce or spinach. Second, go easy on the chicken, potato and macaroni salads (too much mayo). Third, watch your use of shredded cheese. Fourth, top it all off with low-fat dressing.

Reduce the Fat
If you choose lean cold cuts and go easy on the cheese and mayo, your average submarine sandwich is much lower in fat than your typical fast-food fare.

In a Nutshell...

The average fast-food meal is high in fat, calories and salt. It's also lacking in fruits, vegetables and milk products. Limit your intake of high-fat salads, mega burgers, pizza and deep-fried foods. Go for grilled chicken sandwiches and low-fat frozen yogurt or ice milk.

Eighteen

Children and Healthy Eating

Top Ten Things You Should Know about Feeding Your Kids (including the really picky ones)

1. Make Mealtime a Happy Time

Make meals something your kids look forward to. Serve them at the table, fill them with good conversation, and be clear about who is responsible for what. Generally speaking, as a parent your primary concern should be to provide nutritious meals and snacks and serve them at regular, consistent times. Ideally, your children should decide what and how much they eat. In other words, once you put the good stuff on the table, try to relax and let your kids eat as much or as little of each food as they please. The more positive and relaxed the environment, the more food your child is likely to eat. What's more, a relationship based on trust and the division of responsibility helps to positively shape your child's relationship with food later in life.

Get Your Kids to Eat Tip
Kids (and many adults) are more likely to try something if you tell them it tastes good, rather than tell them it's good for them.

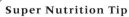

Super Nutrition Tip

Breast milk is the ideal food for infants. Breast milk provides significant protection against gastrointestinal and respiratory illness and may protect against chronic disease and allergies. Infant formula should be used when breast milk is not an option.

Get Your Kids to Eat Tip

At mealtime, try to avoid talking about how much or how little your children are eating. Children should eat to please themselves, rather than to please you. In doing so, they are more likely to stay in touch with their natural hunger cues. They'll eat when they're hungry, they'll stop when they're full.

2. Growing Kids Need Fat

Just because you are trying to eat more low-fat foods doesn't mean your kids need the same. Children need more fat in their diets than adults in order to get the calories and nutrients required for adequate growth and development. This means that during the preschool and childhood years, nutritious food choices like cheese and peanut butter should not be eliminated or restricted because of their fat content. During early adolescence there can be a gradual lowering of fat intake with the understanding that a very active teen will require more fat and calories than an inactive teen. Once a teenager reaches his or her full height (usually mid- to late teens), a diet that includes no more than 30% of energy as fat (the recommended amount of fat for an adult) becomes appropriate. A healthy diet should always be complemented by an active lifestyle.

3. Get Kids Involved

Kids are much more likely to eat a meal when they help in its preparation. Let your kids assist you with meal planning, shopping and food preparation whenever your time and schedule permits. Teach them to cook early on. As they get older have each child responsible for dinner one night of the week. Most kids start to take great pride in their weekly concoction. Once a month have an international night where you feature foods from a foreign country. Make it fun. Put up some decorations, get out a map, and let your kids learn about different cultures from around the world.

4. Keep It Small

When it comes to feeding kids, it's really quite simple. They require the same foods that you do (milk products, grains, fruits and vegetables, meat and alternatives) but in smaller quantities. In general, offer toddlers 1 tablespoon of food for every year of age at each meal. For older children, serve about one half to three quarters of the amount that you would serve yourself. Teenagers, however, depending on their activity level, may well eat significantly more than you. One final tip: when you can, let kids serve themselves. Once again, by feeling more in charge, they feel less pressured to eat and are more likely to eat the foods that are there.

5. Bribery Doesn't Work in the Long Run

To instill a healthy attitude to healthy food, it helps to avoid nagging, coaxing and bribery. Telling your children that they can watch television or have dessert if they eat their vegetables won't make them love veggies. Rather, they will start to think of those foods as "bad" foods or a form of punishment. In one study, two sets of preschoolers were introduced to a new fruit. One group was rewarded for eating the fruit, the other group was not. When the fruit was introduced to both groups a second time, this time with no rewards, the group that had been rewarded the first time around was much less likely to try it again. Even subtle coercion can increase your child's resistance and can interfere with the internal hunger cues that should be guiding his or her appetite.

6. If at First You Don't Succeed, Try, Try Again

Generally speaking, children prefer foods they are familiar with. At the same time, many of the foods children initially reject will be accepted later if the child has ample opportunity to taste the new food. The key word here is "taste." Research tells us that it's not enough for a child to be merely exposed to a food over and over again (although that helps). What really makes the difference is if they actually taste some of it (even a small taste will do). This can be difficult, especially when you are trying to avoid any coaxing or nagging at the table. The

Get Your Kids to Eat Tip
Whenever possible, give your child a choice. For example, ask, "Would you like a banana, an apple or some yogurt for your afternoon snack?" When kids feel in control, they are more likely to accept those foods that are offered.

Super Nutrition Tip
Too many parents think that juice is a low-fat, nutritious alternative to milk. As a result kids are getting so full on fruit juice that there is no room for the nutrients they need for proper growth and development. Most kids should have no more than 1 cup of fruit juice each day, and babies under 1 year, half a cup. Instead of juice, serve fruit some of the time. And make a "milk only" rule at mealtimes since it's milk that kids need more of, not juice.

Super Nutrition Tip
Try to serve desserts that make a contribution on the nutritional front. Foods like low-fat frozen yogurt, fruit salad or applesauce fulfill the need for something sweet while providing a healthy dose of nutrition to boot. In addition, when you serve primarily "healthy desserts" you won't feel so bad on those nights when your child doesn't eat much of the main course. Last but not least, there is no rule that says dessert must be served with every meal.

Get Your Kids to Eat Tip
Don't expect your children to eat much when they are overtired or excited. Don't worry. They'll make up for it the next meal.

trick is to establish, early on, that children taste – just taste, not eat – all new foods. The sooner this expectation is implemented, ideally in late infancy, the more likely it is to be followed without a great deal of trouble. With some kids this is easier than with others. If your child really resists it is better not to force him or her – as they get older most kids will taste new foods more readily. Now comes the next step. Once you get kids to taste new foods on a regular basis, it's time to sit back and wait. It can take as many as eight to ten exposures before a child is truly ready to accept the new food under trial. Unfortunately, most of us give up long before then.

7. The Do's and Don'ts of Snacking

Because they have small tummies, kids need snacks. They are unable to meet their nutritional needs with just 3 meals a day. Plan one nutritious snack between each meal or 2 snacks if meals are spaced farther apart. Ideal snacks include those foods on the Gold snacking list (p.91) – foods like fruits, vegetables, milk, yogurt, cheese and cereal. Discourage children from eating or drinking outside of meal or snacktimes or less than 1 hour prior to mealtime.

> **News Flash: Dieting Is Not for Kids** Children should not be put on a diet. Restricted food intake can affect normal growth and development. The stresses and pressures of dieting can also lead to poor self-esteem, further weight problems and possibly even eating disorders. Instead, children should be provided with healthy food choices and be encouraged to get involved in enjoyable games and physical activities.

8. Don't Be a Short Order Cook

There is no need to be a short order cook in your own kitchen. If you substitute one food for another every time a child doesn't like what you serve, children won't learn to try new foods. If, however, you offer a variety of foods at each meal, a child who won't eat his green beans may still have a bit of chicken, a slice of bread and a glass of milk. And on those nights when your child doesn't want to eat anything at all, don't insist. Just don't give in if your children ask for something to eat 15 minutes after supper's over. They'll have to wait until their regularly scheduled snack time, which may be, for example, shortly before bedtime. Remember, in the end, it's what your child consumes overall that is most important, not what's eaten at each and every individual meal.

Super Nutrition Tip
Your presence at the table means a lot to children. Even if you are not eating, your presence will make them more likely to eat.

> **News Flash: Turn Off the Tube**   Based on a study at the Harvard School of Public Health, a child at a healthy weight who watches 5 or more hours of television a day is 5 times more likely to get fat than a child who watches 2 hours or less.

9. The Potatoes Are Touching the Peas

Having told you there is no need to cater to the food whims and fancies of each child in the family, there are, however, certain areas where a bit of consideration can go a long way. For example, many young children don't like foods touching on the plate, don't like spicy foods, and don't like their foods mixed together. There is no reason not to cater to these preferences. For example, even though you like your chili on the spicy side, you can serve a milder version to your children. With time, most kids will enjoy more spice in their meals. In addition, there is no reason not to cook kids' favourite foods on a regular basis. If Billy loves spaghetti, give him spaghetti. (Just don't give it to him 7 days a week.)

Bottom line: kids are people too, and if you respect some of their likes and dislikes, they feel better about who they are.

10. Kids and Veggies Update

Do you have one of those kids who refuses to eat anything green? Many parents cite vegetables as the number one cause of frustration

Super Nutrition Tip
Don't forget kids need fibre too. To figure out how many grams they need in a day, simply take their age and add the number 5. This rule applies to kids aged 3 to 18. For infants, fibre is also important; however, parents should be careful not to overdo the introduction of high-fibre foods (those containing more than 3 grams of fibre per serving).

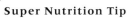

Super Nutrition Tip
What's available in your kitchen cupboards plays a major role in your children's nutritional intake. If your cupboards are filled with Twinkies and Dunkaroos, the fruit bowl will remain untouched. If, however, only healthy options exist, kids quite happily go for the good stuff. And that's not all. If those healthy foods require little or no preparation, they are also more likely to be consumed.

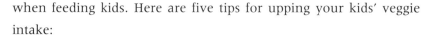

when feeding kids. Here are five tips for upping your kids' veggie intake:

1. Use the blender or food processor to hide vegetables in foods kids love like spaghetti sauce or chili. You can even add pureed carrots to macaroni and cheese.

2. Serve vegetables raw. Most kids prefer them this way. Put a bowl of raw carrot sticks or red pepper slices on the table with most meals and watch how quickly they disappear.

3. Kids love to dip and dunk. Raw veggies and dip are always a hit.

4. Give them vegetables when they're hungry. If your kids are most hungry when they get home from school in the afternoon, have a platter of veggies ready and waiting.

5. While you are getting dinner ready, give your kids some raw veggies to munch on (this is one exception to the no-snacks-before-mealtime rule). With no other foods to compete with, they are more likely to go down.

Kids Are Excellent Food Regulators

One day your kid eats everything on her plate and asks for seconds. The next day she picks at her food and barely makes a dent. Not to worry. Remember two things. First, a child's appetite is often tied to growth spurts. Second, kids are excellent food regulators. In fact, researchers have found that while a child's intake may vary from one meal to the next, most kids are quite consistent in their calorie intake over a 24-hour period. And remember that all kids are unique. For example, your first child might eat everything you put in front of him, while your second child may eat like a bird. Accept and appreciate your children's individual differences. Once again, as long as you provide healthy foods in a pleasant environment, most kids will get what they need.

In a Nutshell...

As a parent you are responsible for providing healthy foods, both meals and snacks, in a positive environment. Your child gets to decide what and how much to eat. Children require regular snacks and smaller portion sizes than adults. Nutritious food choices should not be eliminated or restricted because of their fat content. Have your kids taste new and different foods on a regular basis.

In a Nutshell...

Top Twelve Rules of Healthy Eating

1. *It's Okay to Eat Chocolate*   It's not what you eat at one meal that makes the difference. It's the choices you make overall that are most important.

2. *Small Changes Equal Big Rewards*   A little less butter on your bread, a couple more carrot sticks with your lunch, taking the stairs instead of the elevator: it all adds up to a healthier day.

3. *Eat Less Fat, Especially the Notorious, Artery-Lining Kind*   Your waistline and your heart will thank you for it.

4. *Eat Fruits and Vegetables by the Truckload*   A guaranteed prescription for super health.

5. *Be a Whole-Grain, High-Fibre Feaster*   The absolute foundation of any healthy diet.

6. *Dine on Lean Meats*   Good nutrition with a lot less fat.

7. *Be a Fish Eater*   It's good for your heart.

8. *Say Hello to Beans*   High fibre and super nutrition all in one.

9. *Take a Ride on the Low-fat Milky Way*   Enjoy the wonderful nutrition and bone-building benefits of milk the low-fat way.

10. *Move Your Body*   For health and for happiness, make active living a part of your day.

11. *Take It Slow...One Step at a Time*   Today you may be ready to take the skin off your chicken. Next month you may be ready to try a recipe with beans. Rome wasn't built in a day.

12. *Enjoy Your Food*   Taste it. Savour it. Enjoy each and every bite. Life is meant for living.

The Best of the Best Recipes

Beautiful Breakfasts and Baked Goods   168–172

Sensational Salads and Soups   173–177

Sumptuous Side Dishes and Snacks   178–183

Terrific Turkey and Chicken   184–188

Lean and Tasty Beef and Pork   189–193

Fabulous Fish and Seafood   194–197

Marvellous Meals Without Meat   198–202

Nutritious, Delicious Veggies on the Side   203-208

Delectable Desserts   209–214

Apple Breakfast Bars

These bars are loaded with so much good stuff they put your typical store-bought granola bar to shame.

Makes 20 bars.
Per bar: 137 calories, 4 g fat, 3 g protein, 25 g carbohydrate, 101 mg sodium

1 cup	whole wheat flour	250 mL
3/4 cup	all-purpose flour	175 mL
2/3 cup	packed brown sugar	150 mL
1/2 cup	each chopped dried apricots and prunes	125 mL
1/2 cup	raisins	125 mL
1/4 cup	natural wheat bran	50 mL
1 tsp	baking powder	5 mL
1/2 tsp	cinnamon	2 mL
1/2 tsp	salt	2 mL
1/4 tsp	nutmeg	1 mL
1/4 tsp	baking soda	1 mL
1	apple, grated	1
3/4 cup	plain low-fat yogurt	175 mL
1/4 cup	vegetable oil	50 mL
2	eggs	2

1 In bowl, mix whole wheat and all-purpose flours, sugar, apricots, prunes, raisins, bran, baking powder, cinnamon, salt, nutmeg, baking soda and apple; set aside.

2 Whisk together yogurt, oil and eggs; stir into dry ingredients just until combined. Spread in greased 9-inch (2.5 L) square cake pan.

3 Bake in 350 F (180 C) oven for 35 to 40 minutes or until tester inserted in centre comes out clean. Let cool on rack; cut into bars.

From Canadian Living's Best Light Cooking, *by Elizabeth Baird and the Food Writers of* Canadian Living *Magazine and the* Canadian Living *Test Kitchen (Madison Press Books, 1994).*

Pineapple-Carrot Wheat Muffins

1 1/4 cups	all-purpose flour	300 mL
1/2 cup	wheat germ	125 mL
1/4 cup	oat bran	50 mL
1/2 cup	packed brown sugar	125 mL
1 tsp	baking soda	5 mL
2	eggs	2
1/4 cup	canola oil	50 mL
3/4 cup	buttermilk*	175 mL
1/2 cup	grated raw carrot	125 mL
1	can (8 oz/230 mL) crushed pineapple, drained	1
1 tsp	pure vanilla extract	5 mL

Topping: 1 tbsp (15 mL) wheat germ mixed with 2 tbsp (30 mL) granulated sugar

From more than 500 muffin entries in a contest for healthy eating, this recipe ranked first based on its wonderful taste and outstanding nutritional contribution.

Makes 12 muffins
Per muffin: 178 calories, 6.3 g fat, 101 mg sodium, 1g fibre

1 Preheat oven to 400 F (200 C). Spray 12-cup muffin pan with non-stick cooking spray or line with paper muffin cups.

2 In a large bowl combine flour, wheat germ, oat bran, brown sugar and baking soda.

3 In a separate bowl whisk eggs, oil, buttermilk, carrot, pineapple and vanilla. Add to flour mixture and stir just until dry ingredients are moistened. Divide batter among muffin cups. Sprinkle with topping.

4 Bake 20 minutes or until a toothpick comes out clean. Remove muffins from pan and cool on rack.

* If you do not have buttermilk, substitute sour milk. To make sour milk, place 2 tsp (10 mL) lemon juice or vinegar in a measuring cup and add milk to make 3/4 cup (175 mL). Allow to sit for 10 minutes before using.

Reprinted with permission, Tufts University Diet & Nutrition Letter *(New York, August 1992).*

Apple-Banana Muffins

This recipe received honourable mention in a healthy-eating muffin contest. These muffins are chock-full of good nutrition and simply delicious.

Makes 12 muffins
Per muffin: 194 calories, 5.9 g fat, 126 mg sodium, 2 g fibre

1 cup	all-purpose flour	250 mL
³/₄ cup	whole wheat flour	175 mL
³/₄ cup	old-fashioned oats	175 mL
¹/₄ cup	wheat germ	50 mL
¹/₃ cup	granulated sugar	75 mL
4 tsp	baking powder	20 mL
¹/₂ cup	mashed banana (about 1 large)	125 mL
1	egg	1
¹/₄ cup	canola oil	50 mL
¹/₂ cup	skim milk	125 mL
¹/₂ cup	orange juice	125 mL
¹/₂ cup	diced, unpeeled apple	125 mL
¹/₂ cup	raisins	125 mL

1 Preheat oven to 400 F (200 C). Spray 12-cup muffin pan with non-stick cooking spray or line with paper muffin cups.

2 In a large bowl combine flour, whole wheat flour, oats, wheat germ, sugar and baking powder.

3 In a separate bowl whisk banana, egg, oil, milk and juice. Add to flour mixture and stir just until dry ingredients are moistened. Stir in apple and raisins. Divide batter among muffin cups.

4 Bake 20 minutes or until a toothpick comes out clean. Remove muffins from pan and cool on rack.

Reprinted with permission, Tufts University Diet & Nutrition Letter *(New York, August 1992).*

Make-Ahead Baked French Toast

8	thick slices Italian bread	8
3	eggs	3
1	can (385 mL) Carnation® Evaporated Skim Milk	1
2 tbsp	granulated sugar	25 mL
2 tbsp	frozen orange juice concentrate, thawed	25 mL
1/4 tsp	ground cinnamon	1 mL
	maple syrup	

Thanks to this handy baked version of a breakfast classic, you can relax over orange juice and conversation while family-pleasing French toast crusts to golden perfection.

Makes 4 servings
Per serving without syrup: 312 calories, 4 g fat, 16 g protein, 53 g carbohydrate

1 Place bread slices in single layer in large shallow glass dish.

2 In bowl, beat together eggs, evaporated milk, sugar, orange juice concentrate and cinnamon; pour over bread, turning slices over once. Cover and refrigerate for at least 1 hour or until liquid is absorbed. (Recipe can be prepared to this point and refrigerated for up to 12 hours.)

3 Line jelly roll pan with foil; coat well with nonstick cooking spray. Place soaked bread in single layer on pan; spray each slice with light coating of cooking spray.

4 Bake in 425 F (220 C) oven for 10 minutes. Turn slices over; bake for 5 to 10 minutes or until golden and egg is set. Serve with maple syrup.

From The Best Holidays Ever, *by Nestlé Canada Inc. (Quantum Inc., 1996).*

N.Y.P.D. Blueberry Pancakes

These mouth-watering pancakes won top prize in the "Fabulous Flapjack Flip-off" which took place in New York.

Makes 4 generous servings (8 large pancakes)
Per serving (with topping): 444 calories, 2.2 g fat, 13.9 g protein, 94.3 g carbohydrate, 582 mg sodium

³/₄ cup	whole wheat flour	175 mL
³/₄ cup	all-purpose flour	175 mL
1 tsp	baking powder	5 mL
1 tsp	baking soda	5 mL
1¹/₂ tbsp	sugar	23 mL
2	egg whites	2
1¹/₂ cups	buttermilk	375 mL
¹/₄ cup	low-fat (1% M.F.) cottage cheese	50 mL
¹/₂ tsp	vanilla	2 mL
¹/₄ cup	blueberries	50 mL
	Banana Cream Topping (recipe follows)	
³/₄ cup	pure maple syrup	175 mL

1 In a large bowl, combine flours, baking powder, baking soda and sugar. Set aside.

2 In a medium bowl, whisk together egg whites, buttermilk, cottage cheese and vanilla.

3 Add buttermilk mixture to flour mixture. Stir just until dry ingredients are moistened. Gently stir in blueberries.

4 Spray a large, wide skillet or electric griddle with nonstick spray. Heat over medium heat. For each pancake, spoon about ¹/₂ cup (125 mL) batter onto skillet. Spread to make a 5- or 6-inch circle. Cook until bubbles break through the top and undersides are lightly browned. Flip and cook other side until lightly browned, 2 to 3 more minutes. Serve pancakes topped with 2 tablespoons (30 mL) Banana Cream Topping. Drizzle with maple syrup.

Banana Cream Topping

¹/₂ cup	low-fat sour cream or yogurt	125 mL
¹/₂ cup	mashed banana (about 1 large)	125 mL
2 tbsp	brown sugar	25 mL
¹/₈ tsp	ground cinnamon	.5 mL

1 Combine all ingredients in a small bowl. Cover and refrigerate until ready to use.

From Looneyspoons, *by Janet and Greta Podleski (Granet Publishing Inc., 1996).*

Liz's Poppy Seed Vinaigrette

¼ cup	balsamic vinegar	50 mL
¼ cup	red wine vinegar	50 mL
3 tbsp	sugar	25 mL
1 tsp	Dijon mustard	5 mL
¼ tsp	Worcestershire sauce	1 mL
¼ cup	vegetable oil	50 mL
1 tbsp	poppy seeds	15 mL
2 tbsp	green onions, sliced	25 mL
¼ tsp	paprika	1 mL

This dressing contains half the fat of typical vinaigrette dressings. It is particularly wonderful with dark leafy greens like spinach. Add some sliced strawberries or mandarin orange sections for a sensational salad combination.

Makes 1 cup (250 mL)
Per tbsp (15 mL): 46 calories, 4 g fat, .1 g protein, 3.0 g carbohydrate

1 Combine all ingredients. Mix well. Add to salad just before serving. Dressing can be stored in a glass container in the refrigerator for several weeks.

Herb Buttermilk Dressing

Buttermilk makes a great base for a delicious, low-fat salad dressing.

Makes 1 cup (250 mL)
Per serving (1 tbsp/15 mL dressing):
7 calories, .1 g fat, .5 g protein, .8 g carbohydrate

1 cup	buttermilk	250 mL
1 tbsp	finely chopped fresh dill	15 mL
1 tbsp	finely chopped parsley	15 mL
1 tsp	dried tarragon	5 mL
$1/4$ tsp	Dijon mustard	1 mL
1	small clove garlic, minced	1
$1/2$ tsp	lemon juice	2 mL

1 Combine all ingredients. Refrigerate for up to one week.

From Lucy Waverman's Fast & Fresh Cookbook, *by Lucy Waverman (Firefly Books, 1997).*

Sweet Potato Salad

4	large sweet potatoes	4
	(about 1/2 lb/250g each)	
	Finely grated peel and juice of	
	1 large orange	
2 tbsp	olive oil	25 mL
2 tsp	sesame oil	10 mL
2 tsp	brown sugar	10 mL
2 tsp	Dijon mustard	10 mL
$^1/_2$ tsp	salt	2 mL
$^1/_2$ tsp	pepper	2 mL
	Generous pinch of cayenne pepper	
1	small red onion, finely chopped	1
2 cups	thinly sliced celery	500 mL
$^1/_4$ cup	snipped chives or chopped	50 mL
	fresh coriander	

This is unlike any potato salad you've ever tasted. You'll be asked for the recipe every time you serve it.

Makes 6 to 8 servings
Per serving: 149 calories, 5 g fat, 2 g protein, 26 g carbohydrate, 4 g fibre

1 Sweet potatoes cook quickly, so watch carefully during cooking. If potatoes are overcooked, the salad will be mushy. Slice unpeeled potatoes in half, lengthwise. Place on paper towel in the microwave. Microwave on high until almost fork-tender. Two pounds potatoes (1 kg) will need 10 to 14 minutes. Cover and let stand for 5 minutes. Or bake potato halves in a shallow pan in a 375 F (190 C) oven for 25 to 30 minutes or just until fork-tender. Or cut in half and boil for 20 to 25 minutes.

2 Meanwhile prepare dressing. In a large bowl, whisk orange peel and juice with oils, sugar, Dijon and seasonings. As soon as potatoes are cooked and microwaved potatoes have stood for 5 minutes, run under cold water to stop cooking. Peel potatoes and cut into $^3/_4$-inch pieces. Add warm potatoes to dressing as soon as they are cut. Then, stir in onion, celery and chives. Taste and add more salt and pepper, if needed. Salad is wonderful served warm and can be refrigerated for up to 2 days. Cover, once salad is cold. Bring to room temperature before serving. If salad seems dry, stir in 1 to 2 tablespoons (15 to 30 mL) orange juice or oil. Sprinkle liberally with chives or coriander. Great with chicken.

From The Vitality Cookbook, *by Monda Rosenberg and Frances Berkoff. Copyright © 1995 by Monda Rosenberg and Frances Berkoff. Published by HarperCollins Publishers Ltd. Available at your local bookstore.*

It's Only Brocc 'n Bowl

This cheese and broccoli combination is utterly divine.

Makes 4 to 6 servings
Per serving (based on 6 servings):
109 calories, 3.4 g fat, 8.9 g protein,
13.1 g carbohydrate, 252 mg sodium

1 cup	chopped onions	250 mL
1	clove garlic, minced	1
1/2 cup	chopped celery	125 mL
2 1/2 cups	low-sodium, reduced-fat chicken broth	625 mL
3 cups	broccoli florets	750 mL
1 cup	peeled, cubed potatoes	250 mL
1/2 cup	low-fat sour cream	125 mL
3/4 cup	shredded reduced-fat sharp cheddar cheese	175 mL
1/2 tsp	ground thyme	2 mL
1/2 tsp	black pepper	2 mL
1/2 tsp	"lite" Worcestershire sauce	2 mL
1/4 tsp	salt	1 mL
4–5 dashes	hot pepper sauce	4–5 dashes

Hint
If reheating the soup, don't allow it to boil. The sour cream may cause the soup to curdle.

1 Spray a large saucepan with nonstick spray. Add onions, garlic and celery. Cook and stir over medium heat until celery begins to soften, about 5 minutes. Add broth, 2 cups (500 mL) broccoli and all potatoes. Bring to a boil. Reduce heat to medium-low. Cover and simmer for 10 to 12 minutes, until broccoli and potatoes are tender.

2 While soup is simmering, steam the reserved 1 cup (250 mL) broccoli until tender, about 5 minutes. Set aside.

3 Transfer soup to a blender or food processor, working in batches if necessary. Pulse on and off until soup is coarsely puréed (still kind of chunky). Return puréed soup to pot over low heat. Add reserved steamed broccoli, sour cream, cheese, thyme, pepper, Worcestershire sauce, salt and hot pepper sauce. Stir until smooth. Serve immediately.

From Looneyspoons, *by Janet and Greta Podleski (Granet Publishing Inc., 1996).*

Minestrone Soup

4 cups	vegetable stock	1 L
1 tbsp	olive oil (optional)	15 mL
1 cup	diced carrots	250 mL
1 cup	diced celery	250 mL
1 cup	diced potato	250 mL
$1/2$	large onion, diced	$1/2$
2	cloves garlic, minced	2
2 cups	chopped fresh or canned tomatoes	500 mL
2 tbsp	tomato paste	30 mL
1 tsp	dried basil	5 mL
$1/2$ tsp	dried oregano	2 mL
$1/4$ tsp	celery seeds	1 mL
$1/4$–$1/2$ tsp	salt	1-2 mL
pinch	pepper	pinch
1 cup	sliced zucchini	250 mL
1 cup	green or yellow beans	250 mL
$1/2$ cup	cooked garbanzo, kidney or white beans	125 mL
2 tbsp	chopped parsley	30 mL

Vegetables and beans – could you ask for a more nutritious, delicious combination?

Makes 4 servings
Per serving without oil: 162 calories, 2 g fat, 6 g protein, 35 g carbohydrate, 7 g fibre, 286 mg sodium

1 Sauté carrots, celery, onions and garlic in 2 tbsp (30 mL) of the stock, adding more stock if necessary, or 1 tbsp (15 mL) oil in large pot over medium heat for 5 minutes.

2 Stir in potato, remaining stock, tomatoes, tomato paste, basil, oregano, celery seeds, salt and pepper. Cover, reduce heat and simmer for about 10 minutes or until potatoes are half-cooked.

3 Add zucchini, green beans and your choice of legumes. Cover and cook for about 5 to 7 minutes or until vegetables are tender-crisp. Adjust seasoning and garnish with parsley.

From Cooking Vegetarian, *by Vesanto Melina and Joseph Forest (Macmillan Canada, 1996).*

Beans 'n' Rice

Here's a super recipe to make from scratch or use with rice left over from the night before.

Makes 6 servings
Per serving: 174 calories, 3 g fat, 8 g protein, 28 g carbohydrate, 332 mg sodium

1 tsp	canola oil	5 mL
1	onion, chopped	1
1	clove garlic, chopped	1
1 tsp	chili powder	5 mL
1/2 tsp	ground cumin	2 mL
1/4 tsp	celery seed	1 mL
1/4 tsp	freshly ground pepper	1 mL
1	can (19 oz/540 mL) tomatoes	1
2 cups	cooked red kidney beans	500 mL
1 cup	cooked brown or white long-grain rice	250 mL
1 tsp	Worcestershire sauce	5 mL
1	green sweet pepper, chopped	1
1/2 tsp	salt	2 mL
1/3 cup	shredded cheddar cheese	75 mL
	chopped fresh cilantro or parsley	

1 In large saucepan, heat oil over medium heat; cook onion and garlic, stirring occasionally, for 5 minutes or until onion is translucent. Stir in chili powder, cumin, celery seed and pepper; cook for 1 minute.

2 Add tomatoes, beans, rice and Worcestershire sauce; stir well. Bring to boil, reduce heat and simmer for about 20 minutes or until most of the liquid evaporates.

3 Stir in green pepper. Cook for about 2 minutes or until heated through. Season to taste with salt.

4 Garnish each serving with cheese and cilantro.

From Full of Beans, *by Violet Currie and Kay Spicer (Mighton House, 1993).*

Easy Rice Pilaf Four Ways

4 tsp	butter	20 mL
1	onion, chopped	1
1	clove garlic, minced	1
1 cup	long-grain rice	250 mL
1 1/2 cups	chicken stock	375 mL
1/4 tsp	salt	1 mL
1/4 tsp	pepper	1 mL
2 tbsp	chopped fresh parsley	25 mL

Here are four easy ways to add some life to your rice. Use long-grain brown rice for extra fibre and nutrition.

Makes 4 servings
Per serving: 228 calories, 5 g fat, 6 g protein, 39 g carbohydrate, 478 mg sodium

1 In heavy saucepan, melt butter over medium heat; cook onion and garlic, stirring occasionally, for 3 minutes or until softened. Add rice, stirring to coat.

2 Add chicken stock, salt and pepper; bring to boil. Cover, reduce heat and simmer for 15 minutes or until rice is tender and liquid is absorbed. Fluff with fork. Garnish with parsley.

Variations

Basmati and Red Onion Pilaf   Substitute 1 small red onion, cut into thin strips, for regular onion. Substitute basmati rice for long grain rice. Add 1 bay leaf and 1/4 tsp (1 mL) dried thyme along with rice to pot. Garnish with 1/4 cup (50 mL) toasted chopped cashews along with parsley.

Tropical Pilaf   Add 1 1/2 cups (375 mL) thinly sliced carrots to onion mixture. Cook for 6 to 8 minutes or until almost tender before adding rice. Add pinch each of nutmeg and allspice along with chicken stock.

Italian Pilaf   Add 1/4 tsp (1 mL) dried oregano along with rice. Stir in 1 cup (250 mL) green peas after rice is cooked. Top with 1/4 cup (50 mL) freshly greated Parmesan instead of parsley.

From Canadian Living's Best Light Cooking, *by Elizabeth Baird and the Food Writers of* Canadian Living *Magazine and the* Canadian Living *Test Kitchen (Madison Press Books, 1994).*

Creamy Mushroom Risotto

This dish is laced with wonderful flavour. Be sure to use Arborio or another Italian rice for the perfect creamy texture.

Makes 6 servings
Per serving: 170 calories, 2 g fat, 9 g protein, 29 g carbohydrate

1 $^1/_2$ tsp	olive oil	7 mL
1	onion, chopped	1
2	cloves garlic, finely chopped	2
3 cups	sliced fresh mushrooms (8 oz/250 g)	750 mL
1 $^1/_3$ cups	beef broth	325 mL
$^3/_4$ cup	Arborio or other Italian rice	175 mL
$^3/_4$ tsp	Italian seasoning	4 mL
1	can (385 mL) Carnation® Evaporated Skim Milk	1
2 tbsp	red wine	25 mL
2 tbsp	freshly grated Parmesan cheese	25 mL
	salt and pepper	
	chopped fresh chives or parsley	

Tip
Use a combination of mushrooms if you like – portobello, shiitake, button or porcini.

1 In heavy nonstick saucepan, heat oil over medium-high heat; cook onion and garlic, stirring occasionally, until softened. Add mushrooms; cook, stirring, until moisture is evaporated.

2 Stir in beef broth, rice, Italian seasoning and evaporated milk; cook, stirring, until boiling. Reduce heat to low; cover and cook for 10 minutes, stirring frequently.

3 Uncover and cook, stirring frequently, for 5 minutes longer or until thick and porridge-like. Stir in wine and Parmesan cheese. Add salt and pepper to taste. Serve immediately garnished with chives.

From The Best Holidays Ever, *by Nestlé Canada Inc. (Quantum Inc., 1996).*

Hummus Dip with Tortilla Snackers

Hummus

1	can (19 oz/540 mL) chickpeas, drained	1
1 to 2	cloves garlic, minced	1 to 2
$\frac{1}{2}$ cup	low-fat plain yogurt	125 mL
3 tbsp	lemon juice	45 mL
$\frac{1}{2}$ tsp	salt	2 mL
$\frac{1}{2}$ tsp	ground cumin	2 mL
dash	hot pepper sauce	dash
	freshly ground pepper	

1 In food processor or blender, purée chickpeas with garlic until coarsely chopped. Add yogurt, lemon juice and seasonings; blend to smooth paste.

2 Remove and refrigerate, covered, for at least 2 hours so flavours develop.

Tortilla Snackers

4	8-inch (20 cm) flour tortillas

1 Cut each tortilla with scissors into 12 triangles. Place in single layer on baking pan. Bake in 300 F (160 C) oven for 15 to 20 minutes or until crisp and golden. Allow snackers to cool; store in tightly closed container.

Snacking doesn't get much healthier than this!

Makes 48 tortilla snackers and 2$\frac{1}{3}$ cups (575 mL) hummus.
Per $\frac{1}{3}$ cup (75 mL) hummus with 6 tortilla snackers: 162 calories, 3 g fat, 7 g protein, 28 g carbohydrate, 4 g fibre

From Choice Menus, *by Marjorie Hollands and Margaret Howard (Macmillan Canada, 1993).*

Sun-Dried Tomato and Parsley Pesto Dip

Here's a delicious way to enjoy tofu. Use nutritious dark green and orange vegetables like broccoli and carrots for dipping.

Makes about 2 cups (500 mL)
Per serving (2 tbsp/25 mL): 41.2 calories, 3.2 g fat, 2.1 g protein, 1.4 g carbohydrate

¹/₂ cup	Parsley Pesto (see below)	125 mL
8 oz	soft tofu, drained	250 g
6	drained whole sun-dried tomatoes, packed in oil	6
1	clove garlic, minced	1

1 Using sieve, drain tofu.

2 In food processor and using pulsing motion, combine Parsley Pesto, tofu, tomatoes and garlic; purée until almost smooth.

3 Spoon into serving bowl; cover and refrigerate for up to 2 days.

Parsley Pesto

1 cup	fresh parsley leaves, washed and dried	250 mL
2 tbsp	grated Parmesan cheese (optional, if tolerated)	25 mL
1 tbsp	toasted pine nuts	15 mL
1 tbsp	dried basil	15 mL
1	large clove garlic	1
¹/₂ tsp	salt	2 mL
¹/₄ tsp	black pepper	1 mL
¹/₄ cup	extra virgin olive oil	50 mL

1 In food processor, combine parsley, cheese, pine nuts, basil, garlic, salt and pepper until finely chopped. With motor running, pour in oil. Makes ¹/₂ cup (125 mL).

From The Lactose-Free Cookbook, *by Jan Main (Macmillan Canada, 1996).*

Tortilla Bean Pinwheels

1 cup	cooked kidney beans	250 mL
2 tsp	molasses	10 mL
1 tsp	chili powder	5 mL
1 tsp	Dijon mustard	5 mL
pinch	freshly ground black pepper	pinch
3	8-inch (20 cm) tortillas	3
$^1/_2$ cup	light cream cheese	125 mL
4	green onions, thinly sliced	4

Just one more way to enjoy the goodness of beans.

Makes 9 servings, 36 pinwheels
Per serving (4 pinwheels): 82 calories,
1 g fat, 2 g protein, 10 g carbohy-
drate, 102 mg sodium

1 In small bowl or food processor, mash together or process beans, molasses, chili powder, mustard and pepper until smooth.

2 Spread each tortilla with $^1/_3$ of the cream cheese. Spread bean mixture over cheese. Sprinkle with green onions.

3 Roll up each tortilla, jelly-roll fashion, to make a log. Trim thin ends from each roll. Wrap snugly in plastic wrap or waxed paper. Refrigerate for at least 3 hours or up to 24 hours.

4 At serving time, cut into slices about $^1/_2$-inch (1 cm) thick.

From Full of Beans, *by Violet Currie and*
Kay Spicer (Mighton House, 1993).

Best Ever Turkey Chili

Give this chili a try and chances are you'll be saying it's the best darn turkey chili you've ever tasted.

Makes 4 to 6 servings
Per serving: 234 calories, 3.4 g fat, 24.3 g protein

Lean ground beef or chicken can also be used as an alternative to ground turkey.

1 lb	ground turkey	500 g
1	medium onion, chopped	1
1	clove garlic, minced	1
1/2 cup	chopped celery	125 mL
1	can (28 oz/796 mL) tomatoes	1
1	can (5 1/2 oz/156 mL) tomato paste	1
1 tbsp	Worcestershire sauce	15 mL
1 tbsp	chili powder	15 mL
1 tsp	paprika	5 mL
1 tsp	cumin	5 mL
1	can (19 oz/540 mL) red kidney beans, drained	1

1 In a large heavy saucepan or nonstick skillet, cook turkey over medium-high heat for about 5 minutes. Pour off any fat. Add onion and garlic; cook, stirring, over medium-low heat for 5 minutes or until onions are tender.

2 Add celery, tomatoes, tomato paste, Worcestershire sauce, chili powder, paprika and cumin. Bring to a boil, reduce heat and simmer 20 to 25 minutes, stirring occasionally to break up tomatoes.

3 Add kidney beans, cook 5 minutes longer to heat through.

From Ontario Turkey Producers Marketing Board.

Chicken Dijon

¹/₄ cup	plain yogurt	50 mL
2 to 3 tbsp	Dijon mustard	30 to 45 mL
1 cup	fresh whole wheat breadcrumbs	250 mL
1 tsp	crushed dried thyme leaves	5 mL
¹/₄ tsp	salt	1 mL
¹/₄ tsp	pepper	1 mL
4	skinless chicken breasts or legs (boned if desired)	4

This chicken is too easy and delicious for words. It can be prepared ahead of time and served hot or cold.

Makes 4 servings
Per serving: 178 calories, 3 g fat, 30 g protein, 7 g carbohydrate, 398 mg sodium

1 In small bowl, combine yogurt and mustard. In shallow bowl, mix bread crumbs, thyme, salt and pepper.

2 Spread each piece of chicken with mustard mixture, then roll in breadcrumb mixture. Place chicken in single layer on lightly greased baking sheet.

3 Bake in 350 F (180 C) oven for 45 to 50 minutes for bone-in chicken, 30 minutes for boneless, or until golden brown and meat is no longer pink.

From Smart Cooking, *by Anne Lindsay (Macmillan Canada, 1996).*

Herb-Roasted Chicken Breasts with Garlic, Potatoes and Carrots

This one-dish meal is both delicious and easy to make. I guarantee it will become a family favourite.

Makes 4 servings
Per serving: 454 calories, 10 g fat

2 tbsp	lemon juice	25 mL
2 tbsp	olive oil	25 mL
1/2 tsp	salt	2 mL
1/2 tsp	dried rosmary	2 mL
1/2 tsp	thyme	2 mL
1/4 tsp	pepper	1 mL
12	cloves garlic, peeled	12
1 1/2 lb	small red potatoes, halved	750 g
4	carrots, cut into small chunks	4
1/2 lb	small mushrooms	250 g
4	chicken breast halves	4
1 cup	chicken stock	250 mL

1 Combine lemon juice, oil, salt, rosemary, thyme and pepper; set aside.

2 In large shallow baking dish, toss together garlic, potatoes, carrots, mushrooms and 2 tbsp (30 mL) of the herb mixture; spread out in pan. Arrange chicken, skin side up, on vegetables. Sprinkle with remaining herb mixture. (Can be prepared to this point, covered and refrigerated for up to 1 day; let stand at room temperature for 30 minutes before baking.)

3 Bake uncovered, in upper third of 450 F (230 C) oven for 20 minutes. Reduce temperature to 375 F (190 C). Bake for 25 minutes longer or until chicken is no longer pink inside and vegetables are tender.

4 Transfer chicken and vegetables to heated platter.

5 Add stock to pan and bring to boil, scraping up any brown bits from bottom of pan. Boil until syrupy, about 5 minutes. Pour over chicken and vegetables.

From New Casseroles and Other One Dish Meals, *by Rose Murray (Macmillan Canada, 1996).*

Chicken and Mushroom Burgers

1 lb	lean ground chicken	500 g
1 cup	finely chopped mushrooms	250 mL
	(5 to 6 large)	
$1/2$ cup	chopped onion	125 mL
1	clove garlic, minced	1
$1/4$ cup	fine dried breadcrumbs	50 mL
1 tsp	tarragon	5 mL
$1/4$ tsp	dried thyme	1 mL
$1/4$ tsp	salt	1 mL
$1/4$ tsp	pepper	1 mL
6	whole wheat buns	6

Barbecued or oven broiled, these burgers are sure to be a hit with the whole family. Make extra patties and freeze them for when you need a meal in minutes.

Makes 6 burgers
Per serving: 258 calories, 6 g fat, 22 g protein, 31 g carbohydrate, 3 g fibre

1 In bowl, combine chicken, mushrooms, onion, garlic, breadcrumbs and seasonings. Shape into 6 patties, about $1/2$-inch (1cm) thick.

2 Broil or barbecue for 5 to 6 minutes per side or until brown and chicken is cooked through. Serve on whole wheat buns with garnishes. Suggested garnishes are light mayonnaise, tomato slices, alfalfa sprouts or lettuce, mustard.

From Choice Menus, *by Marjorie Hollands and Margaret Howard (Macmillan Canada, 1993).*

Ten-Minute Make-Ahead Chicken Cacciatore

This recipe has been described as the ultimate weekday entertaining dish. Simply spend 10 minutes the night before getting it ready. All you have to do come dinnertime is put it in the oven.

Makes 6 to 8 servings
Per serving: 185 calories, 2 g fat, 30 g protein, 12 g carbohydrate, 3 g fibre

8	skinless boneless chicken breasts	8
$^1/_2$ lb	large mushrooms	250 g
2	green peppers	2
1	onion	1
1 cup	white wine	250 mL
1	can ($5^1/_2$ oz/156 mL) tomato paste	1
1	can (28 oz/796 mL) tomatoes, well drained	1
4	crushed garlic cloves	4
1 tsp	dried basil or $^1/_4$ cup (50 mL) chopped fresh basil	5 mL
$^1/_2$ tsp	dried leaf oregano	2 mL
1 tsp	salt	5 mL
$^1/_4$ tsp	freshly ground black pepper	1 mL
2	bay leaves	2

1 Place chicken in a lasagna-style dish or casserole that will hold at least 16 cups (4 L). Thickly slice mushrooms. Coarsely chop peppers and finely chop onion. Scatter over and around chicken.

2 Pour wine into a medium-size bowl. Add tomato paste and whisk until evenly blended. Cut tomatoes in half. Stir into wine mixture along with remaining ingredients. Pour over chicken, cover with plastic wrap and refrigerate overnight to allow flavours to blend.

3 When ready to bake, remove casserole dish from refrigerator. Remove plastic wrap and cover with heavy foil. Place in oven and turn heat to 350 F (180 C). Bake for 1 to $1^1/_4$ hours, or until chicken is cooked.

4 Remove chicken to a serving dish. Discard bay leaves. Stir sauce and spoon over chicken. Serve with rotini noodles, rice or couscous.

From The Vitality Cookbook, *by Monda Rosenberg and Frances Berkoff. Copyright © 1995 by Monda Rosenberg and Frances Berkoff. Published by HarperCollins Publishers Ltd. Available at your local bookstore.*

Down Under Beef with Kiwifruit

1 lb	round or sirloin tip steak	500 g

Marinade:

2	ripe kiwifruit, peeled and mashed	2
¼ cup	lime juice	50 mL
¼ cup	water	50 mL
2 tsp	granulated sugar	10 mL
2	cloves garlic, crushed	2
1 tbsp	finely chopped gingerroot	15 mL
1 tsp	dried marjoram	5 mL
½ tsp	freshly ground black pepper	2 mL
2 cups	shell pasta	500 mL
	sliced kiwifruit (garnish)	

Here's a wonderful marinade for lean beef all the way from the land "down under."

Makes 5 servings
Per serving: 256 calories, 3 g fat, 23 g protein, 34 g carbohydrate, 2 g fibre, 35 mg sodium

1 Trim all visible fat from steak and discard.

2 In bowl or plastic bag, combine kiwifruit, juice, water, sugar, garlic, gingerroot and seasonings. Place steak in marinade; refrigerate for about 4 hours to tenderize beef.

3 Remove meat; reserve marinade. Preheat barbecue or broiler on high. Just before cooking brush grill lightly with oil. Broil or barbecue meat 4 inches (10 cm) from heat for about 5 minutes per side, to desired degree of doneness.

4 Meanwhile, in large pot of boiling water, cook pasta according to package directions or until tender but firm; drain well and place in serving dish; keep warm.

5 Slice steak in thin strips. Heat reserved marinade to boiling and pour over cooked pasta. Top with steak strips and serve with kiwifruit garnish.

From Healthy Home Cooking, *by Margaret Howard and Ellie Top (Macmillan Canada, 1993).*

Half Hour Spicy Beef

1 lb	round steak	500 g

Marinade:

2 tbsp	light soy sauce	25 mL
2 tbsp	ketchup	25 mL
2 tbsp	dry sherry OR apple juice	25 mL
2 tsp	minced gingerroot	10 mL
1 tsp	horseradish	5 mL
1 tbsp	vegetable oil, divided	15 mL
2	medium onions, cut into eighths	2
1 cup	cauliflower florets	250 mL
1 cup	broccoli florets	250 mL
3	celery stalks, sliced	3
1	medium zucchini, sliced	1
1/2 cup	carrot coins	125 mL
1/2 tsp	celery seeds	2 mL
1/2 lb	Chinese rice or other noodles	250 g
1/3 cup	low-fat plain yogurt	75 mL

1 Remove all visible fat from beef and discard; cut beef into thin 2-inch (5 cm) strips.

2 In bowl or plastic bag, combine soy sauce, ketchup, sherry, gingerroot and horseradish. Place beef strips in marinade; marinate at room temperature for 20 minutes.

3 In large nonstick skillet, heat 1 tsp (5 mL) oil over medium-high heat; stir-fry onions, cauliflower, broccoli, celery, zucchini, carrot and celery seeds for 6 minutes or until tender-crisp; remove vegetables.

4 Remove beef from marinade; reserve marinade. Add remaining 2 tsp (10 mL) oil to skillet and stir-fry beef for about 3 minutes or until no longer pink. Return vegetables to skillet.

5 Meanwhile, soak rice noodles in boiling water for about 5 minutes (or cook other noodles according to package directions).

6 Drain. Add yogurt to reserved marinade; stir into beef-vegetable mixture and heat briefly. Serve over noodles.

Thirty minutes is all you need – 20 minutes to marinate the beef for exceptional flavour and 10 minutes to cook the meat and vegetables. This recipe works well with whatever vegetables you happen to have on hand.

Makes 6 servings
Per serving: 299 calories, 4.7 g fat, 26 g protein, 40 g carbohydrate, 2.5 g fibre, 615 mg sodium

From Healthy Home Cooking, *by Margaret Howard and Ellie Top (Macmillan Canada, 1993).*

Low-Fat Lasagna

$^1/_2$ lb	lean ground beef	250 g
$^1/_2$ cup	chopped onions	125 mL
$3^1/_2$ cups	chopped tomatoes or	875 mL
1	can (28 oz/796 mL) tomatoes, chopped	1
1	can ($5^1/_2$ oz/156 mL) tomato paste	1
$^1/_3$ cup	Parmesan cheese	75 mL
1 tsp	basil	5 mL
$^1/_2$ tsp	oregano	2 mL
1 tsp	salt	5 mL
$^1/_2$ tsp	pepper	2 mL
3 tbsp	parsley	45 mL
1	cloves garlic, minced	1
6	lasagna noodles	6
8 oz	partly skimmed mozzarella cheese (15% M.F.)	225 g
8 oz	dry curd cottage cheese (1% M.F.)	225 g

Substituting lean ground beef and lower fat cheeses reduces the fat in this family favourite by about 7 grams per serving.

Makes 8 servings
Per serving: 270 calories, 9.8 g fat, 23 g protein, 22 g carbohydrate, 533 mg sodium

1 Preheat oven to 350 F (180 C).

2 Brown beef in heavy pan sprayed with nonstick spray. Remove the meat to a sieve; drain and discard fat. Rinse the pan. Return meat to pan.

3 Add onions, tomatoes, tomato paste, 2 tbsp (30 mL) Parmesan and seasonings. Stir well and simmer at least 30 minutes.

4 Cook lasagna noodles as directed on package, omitting salt. Grate mozzarella cheese. In 7 x 11-inch (18 x 28 cm) pan, layer one third of sauce, 3 noodles and half of each cheese. Repeat, ending with sauce. Bake for 30 to 45 minutes.

From the Beef Information Centre.

Pork Tenderloin with Roasted Sweet Potatoes

This recipe is both incredibly easy to prepare and a guaranteed crowd-pleaser. It comes from a super cook-book designed for families on the go.

Makes 6 servings
Per serving (includes serving ¹/₂ cup/ 125 mL green beans and ¹/₄ cup/50 mL unsweetened applesauce with the pork tenderloin and sweet potatoes): 357 calories, 10 g fat, 27 g protein, 41 g carbohydrate, 6 g fibre

2	pork tenderloins (each about ³/₄ lb/375 g)	2
2 tbsp	honey mustard	25 mL
2 tsp	sodium-reduced soy sauce	10 mL
4	medium sweet potatoes (about 4 , 2 lb/1 kg), peeled and cut into sixths	4
2 tbsp	vegetable oil	25 mL
¹/₄ tsp	pepper	1 mL

1 Preheat oven to 375 F (190 C). Line cookie sheet with foil; lightly grease or spray with nonstick cooking spray.

2 Pat pork tenderloins dry; place in centre of cookie sheet. Combine mustard and soy sauce; brush over top and sides of pork.

3 Pat potatoes dry; toss with oil and pepper. Place around pork.

4 Bake for 40 to 45 minutes or until temperature on meat thermometer registers 160 F (70 C) and potatoes are golden. To serve, slice pork into ¹/₂-inch (1 cm) thick slices.

From Suppertime Survival, *by Lynn Roblin and Bev Callaghan (Macmillan Canada, 1996).*

Shepherd's Pie with Garlic Mashed Potatoes

2 lb	baking potatoes, peeled and cut in 2-inch/5cm pieces	1 kg
12	cloves garlic, peeled	12
³/₄ cup	hot potato cooking liquid or milk	175 mL
	salt and pepper to taste	
1 lb	extra-lean ground beef	500 g
2	onions, chopped	2
2	cloves garlic, finely chopped	2
2 cups	cooked chickpeas, chopped	500 mL
1¹/₂ cups	chili sauce, tomato sauce, ketchup or puréed canned tomatoes	375 mL
1 tbsp	Worcestershire sauce	15 mL
¹/₄ tsp	hot red pepper sauce	1 mL
1 cup	fresh whole wheat or white breadcrumbs	250 mL
¹/₂ cup	fresh or frozen peas	125 mL
¹/₂ cup	fresh or frozen corn niblets	125 mL
1 tbsp	paprika	15 mL

Here's a lighter version of a family favourite. It tastes wonderful and the chickpeas help lower the fat and increase the fibre.

Makes 8 to 10 servings
Per serving: 323 calories, 6 g fat, 20 g protein, 51 g carbohydrate, 8 g fibre, 784 mg sodium

1 Place potatoes and whole garlic cloves in pot and cover with water. Bring to boil and cook for 20 minutes, or until tender. Drain well, reserving about 1 cup (250 mL) cooking liquid. With potato masher or food mill, mash potatoes with ¹/₂ cup (125 mL) hot cooking liquid. Add salt and pepper to taste. Add additional liquid if necessary.

2 Meanwhile, heat large, deep nonstick skillet. Add beef and brown. Add onions and chopped garlic and cook until tender. Drain off any fat if necessary.

3 Add chickpeas and chili sauce. Bring to boil. Reduce heat and cook gently for about 10 minutes.

4 Add Worcestershire, hot pepper sauce, breadcrumbs, peas and corn and combine well. Season to taste with salt and pepper.

5 Transfer mixture to lightly oiled 10 x 8-in. (2.5 L) casserole. Spread or pipe mashed potatoes on top. Dust with paprika. Bake in preheated 400 F (200 C) oven for 30 minutes.

From More HeartSmart Cooking, *by Bonnie Stern (Heart and Stroke Foundation of Canada, Random House Canada, 1997).*

Baked Fish Aegean-style

My daughter calls this tasty fish dish "pizza fish" because of the tomato paste. If you are not a fan of olives, this recipe also tastes great without them.

Makes 4 servings
Per serving: 184 calories, 7 g fat, 22 g protein, 7 g carbohydrate, 169 mg sodium

1 lb	fish fillets (perch, flounder, halibut)	500 g
1 tbsp	dry breadcrumbs	15 mL
2 tbsp	lemon juice	25 mL
$1/4$ cup	tomato paste	50 mL
$1/4$ cup	water	50 mL
2 tsp	extra virgin olive oil	10 mL
1	clove garlic, minced	1
$1 1/2$ tsp	chopped fresh herbs, such as thyme, rosemary, dill and cilantro or $1/2$ tsp (2 mL) dried	7 mL
$1/2$ tsp	ground cumin	2 mL
$1/4$ tsp	crushed red chili pepper flakes	1 mL
$1/4$ tsp	salt and freshly ground black pepper	1 mL
4	pitted black olives, sliced lemon wedges	4

1 With paper towels, pat fish dry.

2 Sprinkle 8-inch (20 cm) square baking dish with breadcrumbs. Arrange fish in single layer on top. Sprinkle with lemon juice.

3 In bowl, combine tomato paste, water, olive oil, garlic, herbs, cumin and chili pepper flakes. Season to taste with salt and pepper. Pour over fish.

4 Bake, uncovered, in 400 F (200 C) oven for 20 minutes or until fish just flakes when touched with fork.

5 Spoon pan juice over fish. Garnish with olive slices and lemon wedges.

Variations

In place of tomato paste mixture, sprinkle fish with $1/2$ tsp (2 mL) paprika, and top with 1 green pepper, sliced, 1 tomato, sliced and 1 small onion, sliced and 1 clove garlic, minced. Drizzle with 2 tsp (10 mL) extra virgin olive oil and season to taste with salt and pepper. Garnish with lemon slices.

From MultiCultural Cooking, *by Kay Spicer (Mighton House, 1995).*

Fish Fillets with Basil and Lemon

1 lb	fish fillets	500 g
1 tbsp	lemon juice	15 mL
2 tsp	margarine, melted	10 mL
$^1/_2$ tsp	dried basil	2 mL
	freshly ground pepper	
	fresh herbs or chopped fresh parsley (garnish)	

Not only is this recipe absolutely marvellous with salmon, when you make it in the microwave it's ready in mere minutes.

Makes 4 servings
Per serving (using cod): 164 calories, 6 g fat, 25 g protein, 0 g carbohydrate, 112 mg sodium

1 In microwave-safe or conventional baking dish, arrange fillets in a single layer. In small dish, combine lemon juice, margarine and basil; drizzle over fish. Sprinkle lightly with pepper to taste.

2 Bake, uncovered, in 450 F (230 C) oven for 8 to 10 minutes (10 minutes per inch thickness of fresh fish) or until fish is opaque and flakes easily with a fork. Sprinkle with fresh herbs or parsley.

Microwave method

Cover with plastic wrap and turn back corner to vent. Microwave at high (100%) power for $3^1/_2$ to $4^1/_2$ minutes or until fish is opaque and flakes easily with fork.

From The Lighthearted Cookbook, *by Anne Lindsay (Key Porter Books, 1988).*

Sesame-Crusted Salmon on Greens

During the week when I'm short on time I often make just the first part of this recipe which involves the salmon. On the weekend, or when I have more time, I make the entire meal – mixed greens, dressing and all. It's incredibly tasty.

Makes 6 servings
Per serving: 242 calories, 10 g fat, 25 g protein, 16 g carbohydrate, 496 mg sodium

6	4 oz (125 g) fillets fresh salmon, skin removed	6
1 tbsp	honey	15 mL
1 tbsp	soy sauce	15 mL
1 tsp	honey-style mustard	5 mL
1 tbsp	sesame seeds	15 mL

Orange Ginger Dressing

1	clove garlic, minced	1
1 tsp	minced fresh gingerroot	5 mL
3 tbsp	orange juice	45 mL
2 tbsp	soy sauce	25 mL
2 tbsp	rice vinegar or balsamic vinegar	25 mL
2 tsp	sesame oil	10 mL
2 tsp	honey	10 mL
1/4 tsp	hot red pepper sauce	1 mL
12 cups	mixed greens	3 L
1 lb	asparagus, trimmed, cooked and cut in 2 inch (5 cm) pieces	500 g
1	sweet red pepper, cut in strips	1
1	orange, peeled and sectioned	1
2 tbsp	chopped fresh cilantro or parsley	25 mL
2 tbsp	chopped fresh chives or green onions	25 mL

1 Pat salmon dry. In small bowl, combine honey, soy sauce and mustard. Rub over salmon. Sprinkle with sesame seeds.

2 Brush nonstick ovenproof skillet lightly with oil. Add salmon and cook for 1 minute per side. Transfer to preheated 425 F (220 C) oven. Cook for 7 to 8 minutes, or until just cooked.

3 To make orange ginger dressing, whisk together garlic, ginger, orange juice, soy sauce, vinegar, sesame oil, honey and hot pepper sauce. Taste and adjust seasonings if necessary. Toss dressing with greens, asparagus, red pepper, orange, cilantro and chives. Serve salad topped with salmon.

From Simply HeartSmart Cooking, *by Bonnie Stern (Heart and Stroke Foundation of Canada, Random House Canada, 1994).*

Shrimp and Garlic Fettuccine Alfredo

12 oz	fettuccine	375 g
1 tsp	olive oil	5 mL
2	cloves garlic, minced	2
½ cup	diced sweet red pepper	125 mL
1	can (385 mL) Carnation® 2% Evaporated Milk	1
¾ cup	(approx) freshly grated Parmesan cheese	175 mL
5 oz	medium shrimp, cooked, peeled and deveined	150 g
½ cup	frozen peas, thawed	125 mL
	salt and pepper	
	chopped fresh parsley (optional)	

Extravagant in flavour but not in fat, here is a lighter version of an all-time favourite. It's sure to draw raves from dinner guests every time you serve it.

Makes 4 servings
Per serving: 508 calories, 12 g fat, 34 g protein, 66 g carbohydrate

1 In large pot of boiling salted water, cook fettuccine for 8 to 10 minutes or until tender but firm; drain well and return to pot.

2 In nonstick skillet, heat oil over medium-high heat; cook garlic and red pepper for 30 seconds or until softened slightly. Add to drained pasta along with evaporated milk and Parmesan cheese. Cook over medium-high heat, stirring gently, for 3 to 4 minutes or until sauce is heated through and thickened slightly.

3 Add shrimp and peas; stir gently until heated through. Remove from heat; let stand for 2 to 3 minutes or until thickened. Season with salt and pepper to taste. Garnish each serving with parsley and additional Parmesan cheese, if desired.

Variations

Classic Fettucine Alfredo   Omit shrimp, red pepper and peas. After sauce has thickened, stir in ¼ cup (50 mL) chopped fresh parsley and season with pinch each of ground nutmeg, salt and pepper.

Alfredo à la Genovese   Substitute 1 cup (250 mL) slivered ham for the shrimp.

From The Best Holidays Ever, *by Nestlé Canada Inc. (Quantum Inc., 1996).*

Bail-Out Bean Burritos

Here you have a nutritious, delicious and easy way to eat more beans. What's more, this meal is especially popular with teens.

Makes 5 servings
Per serving (2 burritos): 528 calories, 14 g fat, 27 g protein, 74 g carbohydrate, 8 g fibre

1	can (14 oz/398 mL) refried beans, lightly mashed	1
1 tsp	chili powder	5 mL
1/2 tsp	ground cumin	2 mL
1/2 tsp	dried oregano leaves	2 mL
1/4 tsp	ground coriander	1 mL
10	8-inch (20 cm) flour tortillas (1 package)	10
1	large tomato, diced (about 8 oz/250 g)	1
2 cups	shredded part-skim mozzarella or cheddar cheese	500 mL
1 cup	prepared salsa	250 mL
1/2 cup	low-fat plain yogurt (2% M.F.)	125 mL
	shredded lettuce (optional)	

1 In microwavable bowl, combine refried beans, chili powder, cumin, oregano and coriander; microwave on medium for 2 to 3 minutes or until heated through. If mixture seems thick, add 1 to 2 tablespoons (15 to 30 mL) water. Place bowl on table. Place tortillas on plate on table.

2 Place tomato, cheese, salsa, yogurt and lettuce (if using) in separate bowls on table.

3 Let people make their own burrito by placing ingredients in centre of tortilla then folding up bottom and sides.

From Suppertime Survival, *by Lynn Roblin and Bev Callaghan (Macmillan Canada, 1996).*

Broccoli Pesto Fettuccine

2 cups	broccoli florets	500 mL
1/2 cup	chopped fresh basil or parsley	125 mL
3 tbsp	olive oil	45 mL
3 tbsp	grated Parmesan cheese	45 mL
3 tbsp	toasted pine nuts	45 mL
1 1/2 tsp	minced garlic	7 mL
1/2 cup	chicken stock	125 mL
12 oz	fettuccine	375 g

Not only is this meal loaded with the goodness of broccoli, the pesto sauce is much lighter than you'd typically find. If you don't have a food processor, use a blender to make pesto sauce.

Makes 6 servings
Per serving: 322 calories, 11 g fat, 11 g protein, 45 g carbohydrates, 3 g fibre, 149 mg sodium

1   Cook broccoli in boiling water or in microwave for 4 minutes, or until tender. Drain and put in food processor along with basil, olive oil, Parmesan, pine nuts and garlic; process until finely chopped. With machine running, add stock through the feed tube; process until smooth.

2   In large pot of boiling water, cook pasta according to package directions, or until tender but firm; drain and place in serving bowl. Pour broccoli pesto over top and toss.

From Enlightened Home Cooking, *by Rose Reisman (Robert Rose Inc., 1996).*

Bruschetta Pizza

If you have yet to try tofu, perhaps I can convince you to try it on pizza.

Makes one 12-inch (30 cm) pizza
Per serving (¹/₆ of pizza): 317 calories, 11.5 g fat, 9.9 g protein, 42.5 g carbohydrate, 1.6 g fibre

1 package	(12 oz/350g) pizza dough	1 package
2 tsp	extra virgin olive oil	10 mL
¹/₂ tsp	dried rosemary	2 mL

Topping

2	large tomatoes, chopped (2 cups/500 mL)	2
¹/₂ cup	chopped red onion	125 mL
¹/₄ cup	chopped fresh parsley	50 mL
2	cloves garlic, minced	2
2 tbsp	extra virgin olive oil	25 mL
2 tsp	dried basil	10 mL
¹/₂ tsp	salt	2 mL

Marinated Tofu (optional)

6 oz	extra firm tofu, crumbled	175 g
1 tbsp	extra virgin olive oil	15 mL
2 tsp	balsamic vinegar	10 mL
1 tsp	dried rosemary	5 mL

grated Parmesan cheese (optional)

1 Preheat oven to 450 F (230 C). Grease 12-inch (30 cm) pizza pan or spray with nonstick baking spray.

2 Marinated Tofu: In mixing bowl, combine tofu, oil, vinegar and rosemary. Let stand about 10 minutes.

3 Meanwhile, roll dough out on floured surface to fit pizza pan. Brush with oil; sprinkle with rosemary. Bake about 5 minutes or until pale brown.

4 Topping: Meanwhile, combine tomatoes, onion, parsley, garlic, oil, basil and salt.

5 Sprinkle partially baked shell evenly with topping and marinated tofu (if using). Bake about 20 minutes or until golden brown on bottom. Remove from oven and sprinkle with Parmesan cheese if tolerated.

From The Lactose-Free Cookbook, *by Jan Main (Macmillan Canada, 1996).*

Penne with Tomatoes, Mushrooms & Basil

1 tsp	olive oil	5 mL
1 cup	sliced mushrooms (about 3 oz/75 g)	250 mL
1	clove garlic, minced	1
5	tomatoes, peeled* and chopped	5
1/3 cup	shredded fresh basil leaves	75 mL
4 cups	small pasta	1 L
	fresh basil sprigs	

Canned tomatoes are an easy substitute for the fresh tomatoes called for in this light-tasting pasta dish.

Makes 6 servings
Per serving: 340 calories, 2 g fat

1 In large nonstick skillet, heat oil over medium-high heat; cook mushrooms and garlic, stirring, 3 to 4 minutes or until softened but not brown.

2 Add tomatoes and basil; reduce heat to medium. Cook, uncovered, 5 minutes.

3 Meanwhile, in large pot boiling salted water, cook pasta 6 to 8 minutes or until al dente (tender but firm). Drain pasta; return to pot over low heat.

4 Add tomato-mushroom mixture; toss well. Spoon into individual pasta bowls; garnish with basil sprigs.

* To peel tomatoes, immerse them in large saucepan boiling water 10 seconds or until skins loosen. Drain then chill under cold running water; remove core and slip off skins.

From Homemaker's Recipe Collection of the Year *(Telemedia Communications Inc., 1993). Recipe by Nancy Enright.*

Tex-Mex Tortilla Pie

Here's a fun way to enjoy tortillas and beans.

Makes 4 servings.
Per serving: 373 calories, 12 g fat, 21 g protein, 50 g carbohydrate, 889 mg sodium

1	can (14 oz/398 mL) beans in tomato sauce	1
1 tbsp	chili powder	15 mL
1/2 tsp	dried oregano	2 mL
1/2 tsp	dried cumin	2 mL
5	8-inch (20 cm) flour tortillas	5
2	fresh or canned jalapeño peppers, finely chopped	2
1 cup	shredded part-skim mozzarella cheese	250 mL
1/2 cup	shredded light cheddar cheese	125 mL

Garnishes

1/2 cup	mild salsa	125 mL
2	medium tomatoes, chopped	2
1/2 cup	shredded lettuce	125 mL

1 In food processor container, process beans and seasonings until smooth.

2 In 9-inch (23 cm) lightly greased baking dish, place 1 tortilla. Spread with one quarter bean mixture, one quarter peppers and one quarter mozzarella. Repeat for 3 more layers. Place last tortilla on top; sprinkle with cheddar.

3 Bake in 350 F (180 C) oven for 20 minutes or until cheese is melted and layers are heated through.

4 Cut into 4 wedges and serve with salsa, tomatoes and lettuce.

From Healthy Home Cooking, *by Margaret Howard and Ellie Top (Macmillan Canada, 1993).*

Butternut Squash Casserole

7 cups	peeled, cubed butternut squash (1 large)	1.75 L
1/2 cup	soft breadcrumbs	125 mL
1/4 cup	coarsely chopped walnuts	50 mL
1/4 cup	chopped fresh parsley	50 mL
1 tbsp	melted soft margarine or butter	15 mL
1/4 tsp	ground nutmeg	1 mL

1 Steam squash over boiling water or microwave in very small amount of water on high (100%) for 10 minutes or until tender; drain well and mash. Lightly spray shallow casserole with nonstick coating; spoon in squash.

2 Combine breadcrumbs, walnuts and parsley. Toss with melted margarine and nutmeg. Sprinkle over squash. Bake in 350 F (180 C) oven for 20 minutes or until hot.

Here's a highly nutritious squash dish. Using the microwave to cook the squash before baking saves both time and energy. Quicker still is the use of frozen squash that's already peeled and cut up.

Makes 8 servings
Per serving: 102 calories, 4 g fat, 2 g protein, 17 g carbohydrate, 1 g fibre, 39 mg sodium

From More Choice Menus, *by Marjorie Hollands and Margaret Howard (Macmillan Canada, 1996).*

Honeyed Carrots

Kids and adults alike will love these sweet-tasting carrots.

Makes 6 servings
Per serving: 109 calories, 3 g fat

1 tbsp	butter	15 mL
1	onion, chopped	1
2 lb	baby carrots, scrubbed	1 kg
1¹/₂ cups	chicken stock	375 mL
1 tbsp	honey	15 mL
¹/₂ tsp	dried thyme	2 mL
2 tbsp	chopped fresh parsley	25 mL

1 In deep skillet, melt butter over medium heat; cook onion, stirring, 2 minutes, until softened.

2 Add carrots, stock, honey and thyme; simmer, uncovered, 20 to 25 minutes, until liquid evaporates and carrots are tender. Stir in parsley before serving.

From Homemaker's *magazine (Telemedia Communications, May 1995). Recipe by Heather Howe.*

Lemon Roasted Potatoes

6	potatoes (unpeeled)	6
2 tbsp	lemon juice	30 mL
1 tbsp	extra virgin olive oil	15 mL
2 tbsp	chopped fresh parsley	30 mL
1 tsp	dried basil	5 mL
1/2 tsp	dried oregano	2 mL
1/2 tsp	salt	2 mL
1/4 tsp	pepper	1 mL

This recipe is simply fabulous. What's more, it works equally well with carrots or sweet potatoes.

Makes 6 servings
Per serving: 155 calories, 2 g fat, 3 g protein, 31 g carbohydrate, 3 g fibre, 188 mg sodium

1 Wash potatoes and cut each into eight. Toss in large bowl with lemon juice, olive oil, parsley, basil, oregano, salt and pepper.

2 Transfer to 13 X 9-inch (3 L) baking dish and bake, uncovered in 350 F (180 C) oven for 30 minutes or until soft.

From Cooking Vegetarian, *by Vesanto Melina and Joseph Forest (Macmillan Canada, 1996).*

Modern Mashed Potatoes

4	large potatoes	4
4	large, whole unpeeled garlic cloves	4
1/2 to 2/3 cup	buttermilk or light sour cream	125mL to 150 mL
	salt and ground white pepper	

The first time I made this recipe was at a family Thanksgiving dinner. It was such a hit I now make it on a regular basis. By the way, this cookbook is filled with great ideas on how to add more fruits and vegetables to your diet.

Makes 4 servings
Per serving: 172 calories, trace of fat, 5 g protein, 38 g carbohydrate, 3 g fibre

1 Cut unpeeled potatoes in half. Place in a saucepan with garlic and about 1/2 teaspoon (2 mL) salt. Generously cover with warm water and bring to a boil. Then, adjust heat and boil gently until potatoes are very soft, about 30 to 40 minutes.

2 Drain potatoes and garlic. Peel and place in a mixing bowl. (Don't do this in a food processor or you'll make glue.) Peel whole garlic cloves and add. Mash garlic with a fork. Then, mash potatoes with a potato masher. Using a spoon or electric mixer, gradually whip in 1/4 cup (50 mL) buttermilk. Then, continue adding the milk, 1 to 2 tablespoons (15 mL to 30 mL) at a time, just until light and creamy. Add salt and white pepper as needed. Serve immediately.

From The Vitality Cookbook, *by Monda Rosenberg and Frances Berkoff. Copyright © 1995 by Monda Rosenberg and Frances Berkoff. Published by HarperCollins Publishers Ltd. Available at your local bookstore.*

Spicy Mashed Sweet Potatoes

6	large sweet potatoes (3 lb/1.5 kg)	6
1	baking potato ($^1/_2$ lb/250g)	1
3 tbsp	brown sugar or honey	45 mL
$^1/_2$ tsp	pepper	2 mL
$^1/_2$ tsp	cayenne (more or less to taste)	2 mL
pinch	nutmeg	pinch
	salt to taste	

Here's a tasty way to serve nutritious sweet potatoes. This is a spicy version. Try the maple variation below if you prefer sweet sweet potatoes.

Makes 6 to 8 servings
Per serving: 191 calories, trace fat, 3 g protein, 46 g carbohydrate, 5 g fibre, 17 mg sodium

1 Prick potatoes and place on baking sheet. Bake in preheated 350 F (180 C) oven for 1 hour, until very tender when pierced.

2 Spoon potatoes out of their skins into bowl or food mill.

3 Mash potatoes with sugar, pepper, cayenne, nutmeg and salt. Taste and adjust seasonings if necessary.

Maple Mashed Sweet Potatoes

Use maple syrup instead of brown sugar. Omit cayenne. Add $^1/_2$ tsp (2 mL) cinnamon and pinch allspice.

From More HeartSmart Cooking, *by Bonnie Stern (Heart and Stroke Foundation of Canada, Random House Canada, 1994).*

Sunflower Seed and Orange Broccoli

This recipe is a delicious answer to the call to eat more vegetables. Even more exciting, it's made with the nutritious all-star, broccoli.

Makes 6 servings
Per serving: 57 calories, 4 g fat, 2 g protein, 4 g carbohydrate, 2 g fibre

1	bunch broccoli, cut into florets	1
2 tbsp	orange juice	25 mL
2 tsp	lemon juice	10 mL
1 tbsp	vegetable oil	15 mL
$1\frac{1}{2}$ tsp	granulated sugar	7 mL
$\frac{1}{2}$ tsp	crushed dried basil	2 mL
$\frac{1}{4}$ tsp	coarsely ground black pepper	1 mL
$\frac{1}{4}$ tsp	Dijon mustard	1 mL
2 tbsp	unsalted shelled sunflower seeds	25 mL

1 In saucepan of boiling water, blanch broccoli for 2 minutes or until tender-crisp. Drain and refresh in cold water; set aside.

2 In small bowl, combine orange and lemon juices, oil, sugar, basil, pepper and mustard; whisk until blended. In nonstick skillet lightly coated with vegetable oil spray, toast sunflower seeds over medium heat.

3 In skillet, drizzle broccoli with juice mixture; cover and heat 3 to 5 minutes or until heated through. Sprinkle with sunflower seeds.

From Healthy Pleasures, *by the Canadian Dietetic Association in collaboration with the Canadian Federation of Chefs and Cooks (Macmillan Canada, 1995).*

Apple Cranberry Clafoutis

1 tbsp	margarine or butter	15 mL
6 cups	sliced baking apples	1.5 L
½ cup	fresh or frozen cranberries	125 mL
½ cup	low-fat milk	125 mL
⅓ cup	all-purpose flour	75 mL
⅓ cup	granulated sugar	75 mL
3	eggs	3
1 tbsp	rum or brandy or 1 tsp (5 mL) rum or brandy extract	15 mL
¼ tsp	baking powder	1 mL
2 tbsp	granulated sugar	25 mL
1 tsp	ground cinnamon	5 mL

Here's a great recipe made with the goodness of fruit.

Makes 6 servings
Per serving: 223 calories, 5.2 g fat, 4.8 g protein, 40 g carbohydrate, 2.8 g fibre, 75 mg sodium

1 In large microwavable container, microwave margarine at high (100%) for 20 seconds or until melted. Stir in apples and microwave at high for 4 minutes or until apples are barely tender. Stir in cranberries; turn into 10-inch (25 cm) quiche dish.

2 In blender container or small bowl, blend milk, flour, ⅓ cup (75 mL) sugar, eggs, rum and baking powder until well combined. Pour over apple mixture.

3 Combine 2 tbsp (30 mL) sugar and cinnamon; sprinkle over top of clafoutis. Bake in 350 F (180 C) oven for 45 minutes or until puffed and set. Cut into wedges and serve warm.

From Healthy Home Cooking, *by Margaret Howard and Ellie Top (Macmillan Canada, 1993).*

Blueberry Strawberry Pear Crisp

The great thing about "crisps" is not only their taste, but also the fact that you can make them with whatever combination of fruits you happen to have on hand. This combination is particularly delicious.

Makes 8 servings
Per serving: 267 calories, 5 g fat, 3 g protein, 54 g carbohydrates, 3 g fibre, 69 mg sodium

1 1/2 cups	fresh blueberries (or frozen, thawed and drained)	375 mL
1 1/2 cups	sliced strawberries	375 mL
1 1/2 cups	chopped peeled pears	375 mL
1/2 cup	granulated sugar	125 mL
2 tbsp	all-purpose flour	25 mL
2 tsp	orange juice	10 mL
1 tsp	grated orange zest	5 mL
1/2 tsp	cinnamon	2 mL

Topping

3/4 cup	brown sugar	175 mL
3/4 cup	all-purpose flour	175 mL
1/2 cup	rolled oats	125 mL
1/2 tsp	cinnamon	2 mL
1/4 cup	cold margarine or butter	50 mL

1 In a large bowl, combine blueberries, strawberries, pears, sugar, flour, orange juice, orange zest and cinnamon; toss gently to mix. Spread in 9-inch (2.5 L) square cake pan.

2 In small bowl, combine brown sugar, flour, oats and cinnamon; cut margarine in until crumbly. Sprinkle over fruit mixture. Bake in 350 F (180 C) oven for 30 to 35 minutes or until topping is browned and fruit is tender.

From Enlightened Home Cooking, *by Rose Reisman (Robert Rose Inc., 1996).*

Buttermilk Oat-Branana Cake

1 cup	buttermilk	250 mL
2/3 cup	rolled oats	150 mL
1/3 cup	oat bran or wheat bran	75 mL
1/4 cup	butter or margarine	50 mL
1 cup	granulated sugar	250 mL
1	egg	1
1 tsp	vanilla extract	5 mL
2	ripe bananas, mashed	2
1 1/2 cups	all-purpose flour	375 mL
1 tsp	baking soda	5 mL
1 tsp	baking powder	5 mL

Glaze

1/2 cup	granulated sugar	125 mL
1/2 cup	buttermilk	125 mL
1/4 cup	butter or margarine	50 mL
1/2 tsp	baking soda	2 mL

This fabulous cake got honourable mention in a healthy eating contest. It's both nutritious and delicious – who could ask for more?

Makes 8 generous servings or 12 smaller servings
Per serving: 277 calories, 8.8 g fat, 4.5 g protein, 46.3 g carbohydrate, 1.5 g fibre

1 In small bowl, pour buttermilk over rolled oats and oat bran. Let stand for 10 minutes.

2 In medium bowl, cream butter and sugar. Beat in egg and vanilla. Combine bananas and buttermilk-oat mixture with creamed ingredients. Sift together flour, baking soda and baking powder. Stir dry ingredients into banana mixture; blend well.

3 Pour batter into lightly greased and floured 8-inch (2 L) square cake pan. Bake in 350 F (180 C) oven for 45 minutes, or until tester inserted in centre comes out clean. Let stand 5 minutes.

4 Meanwhile, prepare glaze. In small saucepan over medium heat, combine sugar, buttermilk, butter and baking soda. Bring just to boil. (Watch closely, mixture will foam.) Makes approximately 2 cups (500 mL) glaze.

5 Poke holes with tester (a metal skewer or a wooden toothpick) all over cake surface; pour glaze over cake while still warm. Cool cake before cutting.

From Eat Well, Live Well, *by Helen Bishop MacDonald and Margaret Howard (Macmillan Canada, 1990).*

Fresh Plum Flan

Anne Lindsay is one of the top cook-book authors in the country for good reason. Here is one of her favourite recipes.

Makes 10 servings
Per serving: 222 calories, 6 g fat, 3 g protein, 40 g carbohydrate, 1 g fibre, 106 mg sodium

Please note
This recipe can also be made with canned plums (two 14 oz/398 mL cans are required).

³/₄ cup	granulated sugar	175 mL
¹/₄ cup	soft margarine or butter	50 mL
2	eggs	2
1 cup	all-purpose flour	250 mL
1 tsp	baking powder	5 mL
1 tsp	grated orange or lemon rind	5 mL
¹/₄ cup	low-fat milk	50 mL
2 cups	halved pitted plums	500 mL
¹/₂ cup	packed brown sugar	125 mL
1 tsp	cinnamon	5 mL

1 In large bowl and using electric mixer, cream together granulated sugar and margarine; beat in eggs one at a time, beating well after each addition.

2 Combine flour, baking powder and orange rind; beat into egg mixture alternately with milk, making three additions of flour and two of milk.

3 Turn into greased 10-inch (3 L) springform pan. Arrange plums, cut side down, in circles on top, lightly pushing into batter.

4 Combine brown sugar and cinnamon; sprinkle over plums. Bake in 350 F (180 C) oven for 45 to 55 minutes or until top is golden and toothpick inserted into flan comes out clean.

Variations

Fresh Apple Flan   Instead of plums, use 2 large apples, peeled, cored and cut into ¹/₄-inch (5 mm) thick slices. Arrange slightly overlapping slices in circles on top, lightly pushing into batter.

From Anne Lindsay's Light Kitchen, *by Anne Lindsay (Macmillan Canada, 1994).*

Say "Cheesecake"

1 $^1/_2$ cups	crushed low-fat graham wafers	375 mL
1 tbsp	sugar	15 mL
1	egg white	1
1 cup	low-fat (1% M.F.) cottage cheese	250 mL
2 cups	low-fat sour cream	500 mL
$^1/_2$ cup	sugar	125 mL
2 tbsp	all-purpose flour	25 mL
1	egg	1
2	egg whites	2
2 tsp	vanilla	10 mL
1	can (19 oz/540 mL) cherry or blueberry pie filling, or fresh fruit to top cake	1

It's hard to believe that this mouth-watering cheesecake has just over 3 grams of fat per serving. By the way, if you're looking for a fun cookbook, nothing could be more fun than this one.

Makes 8 large servings
Per serving: 281 calories, 3.6 g fat, 11 g protein, 53.7 g carbohydrate, 234 mg sodium

1 Preheat oven to 375 F (190 C).

2 Spray an 8-inch (20 cm) springform pan with nonstick spray. Set aside.

3 In a small bowl, mix together graham crumbs and sugar. Add egg white. Stir until well blended. Press crumb mixture firmly over bottom and part way up sides of springform pan. Bake just until edges feel firm and dry, about 8 minutes. Be careful not to overbake. Set aside to cool. Reduce oven to 300 F (150 C).

4 In blender, process cottage cheese and sour cream until smooth (about 1 minute). Add sugar, flour, egg, egg whites and vanilla and process again until well blended.

5 Pour filling into pie crust and bake about 1 hour and 15 minutes, or until edges are dry to touch and centre jiggles only slightly when pan is shaken. Remove from oven and cool completely. Cover and refrigerate for at least 5 hours before serving. Run a knife along inside edge of pan and remove sides. Serve with pie filling or fresh fruit on top.

From Looneyspoons, *by Janet and Greta Podleski (Granet Publishing Inc., 1996).*

Strawberry Cream Mould

Light is the operative word for this
luscious dessert, which is similar to
a Spanish or Bavarian cream.

Makes 6 servings
Per serving: 117 calories, 3 g fat, 4 g
protein, 19 g carbohydrate, 76 mg
sodium

¹/₂ cup	water	125 mL
1	package low-calorie strawberry jelly powder	1
¹/₂ cup	ice cold water	125 mL
2 cups	low-calorie dessert topping	500 mL
2	egg whites, beaten	2
1 cup	sliced fresh or frozen strawberries	250 mL

1 Boil water; stir in strawberry gelatin until dissolved. Stir in cold water. Refrigerate for about 15 minutes or until partially set. Prepare dessert topping. Fold into gelatin until smooth. Chill for 15 minutes.

2 Beat egg whites until stiff peaks form. Fold into strawberry gelatin mixture. Set aside 12 strawberry slices for garnish. Fold remaining strawberries into gelatin mixture. Pour into ring mould.

3 Cover and chill in refrigerator for 4 hours or until firm.

4 Unmould onto serving plate. Garnish with reserved strawberry slices.

From MultiCultural Cooking, *by Kay*
Spicer (Mighton House, 1995).

Summary of Key References

Fats

Caggiula, A., and Mustad, V. "Effects of dietary fat and fatty acids on coronary artery disease risk and total lipoprotein cholesterol concentrations: Epidemiologic studies." *American Journal of Clinical Nutrition* 65 (1997, supplement): 1597–610.

Jonnalagadda, S., et al. "Effects of individual fatty acids on chronic diseases." *Nutrition Today* 31 (May/June 1996): 90–107.

Kristal, A., et al. "Long-term maintenance of a low fat diet: Durability of fat-related dietary habits in the Women's Health Trial." *Journal of The American Dietetic Association* 92 (May 1992): 553–59.

Schaefer, E. "Effects of dietary fatty acids on lipoproteins and cardiovascular disease risk: Summary. "*American Journal of Clinical Nutrition* 65 (1997, supplement): 1655–56.

Smith-Schneider, L., et al. "Dietary fat reduction strategies." *Journal of the American Dietetic Association* 92 (January 1992): 34–8.

Fruits & Vegetables

American Dietetic Association. "Position of The American Dietetic Association: Phytochemicals and functional foods." *Journal of the American Dietetic Association* 95 (April 1995): 493–96.

Harvard University. "Pesticide residues: Forbidden fruit?" *Harvard Health Letter* (January 1994): 6–7.

Steinmetz, K., and Potter, J. "Vegetables, fruit, and cancer prevention: A review." *Journal of the American Dietetic Association* 96 (October 1996): 1027–39.

Williamson, G. "Protective effects of fruits and vegetables in the diet." *Nutrition & Food Science* 1 (January/February 1996): 6–9.

Grains

Glore, S., et al. "Soluble fiber and serum lipids: A literature review." *Journal of the American Dietetic Association* 94 (April 1994): 425–35.

Slavin, J. *Fibre Update*. Kellogg Canada Inc. 1995.

Slavin, J. "Whole grains and health: Separating the wheat from the chaff." *Nutrition Today* 29 (July/August 1994): 6–11.

Smallwood, D., and Blaylock, J. "Fiber: Not enough of a good thing?" *Food Review* (January/April 1994): 23–9.

Beef/Chicken/Pork

Chambers, E. "The skinny on cooking chicken." *Journal of the American*
Dietetic Association 95 (February 1995): 167.

National Institute of Nutrition. "Making the best use of family food expenditure data." *Rapport* 11 (Spring 1996): 1, 6–7.

Nicklas, T. "Impact of meat consumption on nutritional quality and cardiovascular risk factors in young adults: The Bogalusa Heart Study." *Journal of the American Dietetic Association* 95 (August 1995): 887–92.

Fish

Harris, W. "n-3 fatty acids and serum lipoproteins: Human studies." *American Journal of Clinical Nutrition* 65 (1997, supplement): 1645–54.

Nettleton, J. "Omega-3 fatty acids: Comparison of plant and seafood sources in human nutrition." *Journal of the American Dietetic Association* 91 (March 1991): 331–6.

Schardt, D., and Schmidt, S. "Fishing for safe seafood." *Nutrition Action Health Letter* 23 (November 1996): 1, 3–5.

Eggs

Howell, W. "Diet and blood lipids." *Nutrition Today* 32 (May/June 1997): 110–115.

Retzlaff, B., et al. "Effects of two eggs per day versus placebo in moderately hypercholesterolemic and combined hyperlipidemic subjects consuming the NCEP Step-One Diet." *Circulation* 92 (Oct. 1995).

Beans

American Institute for Cancer Research. "More than a hill of beans." *Newsletter* 49 (Fall 1995): 10–11.

Dwyer, J., et al. "Tofu and soy drinks contain phytoestrogens." *Journal of the American Dietetic Association* 94 (July 1994): 739–43.

Mayo Clinic. "Soy: A healthful diet addition." *Health Letter* (May 1997): 7.

Nuts

Dreher, M., et al. "The tradition and emerging role of nuts in healthful diets." *Nutrition Reviews* 54 (August 1996): 241–45.

University of California at Berkeley. "Nuts to you." *Wellness Letter* 13 (February 1997): 3.

Milk Products

"Consensus statements from the Scientific Advisory Board of the Osteoporosis Society of Canada." *Canadian Medical Association Journal* 155 (October 1996).

Hertzler, S., et al. "How much lactose is low lactose?" *Journal of the American Dietetic Association* 96 (March 1996): 243–6.

Jenkins, E., and Jones, C. "It pays to look after your bones!" *Nutrition & Food Science* 1 (January/February 1996): 14–19.

National Institute of Nutrition. The Role of Dairy Products in the Canadian Diet. July 1995.

Vegetarianism

Janelle, C., and Barr, S. "Nutrient intakes and eating behavior scores of vegetarian and nonvegetarian women." *Journal of the American Dietetic Association* 95 (February 1995): 180–8.

Mayo Clinic. "Vegetarian diets." *Health Letter* (January 1995): 7.

University of California. "The effects of vegetarian diets on infants and children." *Nutrition & the M.D.* 22 (August 1996): 6–7.

University of California. "Vegetarian diets: Nutrients and diet." *Nutrition & the M.D.* 22 (August 1996): 1–2.

Snacking/Desserts

Cross, A., et al. "Snacking patterns among 1,800 adults and children." *Journal of the American Dietetic Association* 94 (December 1994): 1398–1403.

Ferguson, K. "Characteristics of successful dieters as measured by guided interview responses and Restraint Scale scores." *Journal of the American Dietetic Association* 92 (September 1992): 1119–20.

Water

Canada. Health and Welfare Canada, Health Protection Branch. *Drinking Water Guidelines.* Ottawa: Ministry of Supply and Services Canada, March 1994.

City of Toronto Department of Public Health. The quality of drinking water in Toronto: A review of tap water, bottled water and water treated by a point-of-use device. *Summary Report* (December 1990).

International Bottled Water Association. *International Bottled Water Association Model Bottled Water Regulation.* March 1995.

Levine, B. "Most frequently asked questions...about water." *Nutrition Today* 31 (September/October 1996): 209–10.

Coffee

International Food Information Council. "Caffeine and health: Clarifying the controversies." *IFIC Review* (May 1993).

Papadopoulos, S. "Coffee, caffeine and health: The real story." *Nutrition & Food Science* 1 (January/February 1993): 28–33.

Tea

Kell, S., et al. "Dietary flavonoids, antioxidant vitamins and incidence of stroke." *Archives of Internal Medicine* 156 (March 1996): 637–42.

University of California. "Chinese green tea: Can it prevent cancer?" *Nutrition & the M.D.* 21 (February 1995): 7.

Zheng, W., et al. "Tea consumption and cancer incidence in a prospective cohort study of postmenopausal women." *American Journal of Epidemiology* 144 (1996): 175–81.

Alcohol

Ashley, M., et al. "Moderate drinking and health: Report of an international symposium." *Canadian Medical Association Journal* 151 (September 1994): 809–25.

Jacyk, W. "Moderate drinking and health: proceedings of an international conference". *Canadian Medical Association Journal* 161 (September 1994): 748–50.

Tufts University. "Seven questions and answers about the diet-cancer connection." *Diet and Nutrition Letter* 14 (December 1996): 5.

Sugar/Sugar Substitutes

American Dietetic Association. "Position of The American Dietetic Association: Use of nutritive and nonnutritive sweeteners." *Journal of the American Dietetic Association* 93 (July 1993): 816–20.

Wolraich, M., et al. "Effects of diets high in sucrose or aspartame on the behavior and cognitive performance of children." *New England Journal of Medicine* 330 (February 1994): 301–7.

Salt

Cutler, J., et al. "Randomized trials of sodium reduction: An overview." *American Journal of Clinical Nutrition* 65 (1997, supplement): 643–51.

Stamler, J. "The INTERSALT Study: Background, methods, findings, and implications." *American Journal of Clinical Nutrition* 65 (1997, supplement): 626–42.

University of California. "A perspective on reducing salt intake." *Nutrition & the M.D.* 22 (March 1996): 5, 8.

University of California at Berkeley. "Don't let the salt news shake you up." *Wellness Letter* 12 (September 1996): 1–2.

Weight Control

American Dietetic Association. "Position of the American Dietetic Association: Weight management." *Journal of the American Dietetic Association* 97 (January 1997): 71–74.

Committee to Develop Criteria for Evaluating the Outcomes of Approaches to Prevent and Treat Obesity. "Summary: Weighing the options-Criteria for evaluating weight-management programs." *Journal of the American Dietetic Association* 95 (January 1995): 96–105.

Conferences, Symposia and Reports. "Obesity solutions: The next decade coping with an epidemic." *Nutrition Today* 31 (July/August 1996): 173–74.

Kratina, K., and King, N. "Hunger and satiety: helping clients get in touch with body signals." *Healthy Weight Journal* 4 (July/August 1996): 68–71.

Parham, E. "Is there a new weight paradigm?" *Nutrition Today* 31 (July/August 1996): 155–61.

Robison, J., et al. "Redefining success in obesity intervention: The new paradigm." *Journal of the American Dietetic Association* 95 (April 1995): 422–24.

Surgeon General's Report. "Summary of the Surgeon General's Report addressing physical activity and health." *Nutrition Reviews* 54 (September 1996): 280–84.

Vitamin & Mineral Supplements

American Dietetic Association. "Position of The American Dietetic Association: Vitamin and mineral supplementation." *Journal of the American Dietetic Association* 96 (January 1996): 73–7.

Gaziano, M. "Antioxidants in cardiovascular disease: Randomized trials." *Nutrition Reviews* 54 (June 1996): 175–84.

National Institute of Nutrition. "Nutraceuticals." *Rapport* 11 (Winter 1996): 1–6.

Thomas, P. "Food for thought about dietary supplements." *Nutrition Today* 31 (March/April 1996): 46–54.

Convenience/Dining Out/Fast Food

Canadian Foundation for Dietetic Research. *Speaking of Food and Eating.* 1997.

Castro, J. "Social facilitation of food intake: People eat more with other people." *Food & Nutrition News* 66 (1994): 29–30.

KFC Nutritional Information (December 1996).

McDonald's Food Facts (September 1996).

Pizza Hut Nutritional Information (October 1994).

Swiss Chalet's Guide To Good Eating (May 1995).

Wendy's Nutrition Guide (November 1995).

Feeding Your Kids

Birch, L. "Children's food acceptance patterns." *Nutrition Today* 31 (November/December 1996): 234–40.

Canada. Health Canada. *Food For Thought: An Exploratory on Children and Healthy Eating.* Ottawa: Ministry of Supply and Services Canada, 1996.

Glinsmann, W., et al. "Dietary guidelines for infants: A timely reminder." *Nutrition Reviews* 54 (February 1996): 50–7.

Johnson, D. "Nutrition in infancy: Evolving views on recommendations." *Nutrition Today* 32 (March/April 1997): 63–8.

Nutrient Data

Brault Dubuc, M., and Caron Lahaie, L. *Nutritive Value of Foods.* 2nd edition. Société Brault-Lahaie. 1994.

Canada. Health and Welfare Canada. *Nutrient Value of Some Common Foods.* Ottawa: Ministry of Supply and Services Canada, 1988.

Manufacturers' product labels

Pennington, J. *Bowes and Church's Food Values of Portions Commonly Used.* 15th edition. HarperPerennial. 1989.

Liz Pearson is an award-winning professional speaker who conducts seminars for corporations, associations, health professionals and the general public. Her clients include companies such as IBM, Hoffman La-Roche, and Warner-Lambert.

If you would like to book or receive information on any of Liz's seminars, please contact:

The Pearson Institute of Nutrition

Telephone: 416-759-4823

Fax: 416-759-7842

E-mail: LizPearson@aol.com

Web site: http://members.aol.com/LizPearson

Index

added fats, 14

air travel:
   and food, 150–1; and water, 151

alcohol:
   benefits, 110–11; and breast cancer, 112–13; calories, 114; grams of fat, 114; and water, 102

allergies, peanut butter, 71

allium vegetables, and phytochemicals, 20

antibiotics, in food supply, 48–9

antioxidants, 19–20, 111, 140

artery-lining fat. *See* saturated fats

bagels, 37

beans, 61–7
   dips, 91; fat content, 61–2; serving suggestions, 65–7, 144

beef:
   cooking tip, 47; grams of fat, 46; ground, 44, 47

The Best of the Best Recipes index, 220

beta-carotene, 18, 19, 137, 140

blood cholesterol level:
   reduced with soy products, 63; and saturated fat, 7–8, 57
   See also cholesterol

blood sugar control, 32
   and snacking, 86; soluble fibre, 31

body fat, excess, 126

body image, unrealistic, 131, 134

Body Mass Index (BMI), 127

bone health, 73–4

breads, 35, 91

breakfast:
   cereals and, 37; fast food, 154

breast cancer:
   and alcohol, 112–13; insoluble fibre, 31; and soybeans, 62

breast milk, 157, 158
   fat content, 14

broccoli, 20–1

butter, 13

grams of fat, 36, 77; and margarine, 11

buttermilk, 79

cabbage, 20

caffeine, 105–7
   and children, 106–7; content, 107

calcium, 137, 140
   and bone health, 73–4; daily requirement, 80; sources, 77; supplements, 80, 82

calories, 128
   daily requirement, 13–14; from fat, 9; per gram, 8

cancer:
   and alcohol, 112; and antioxidants, 19; and CLA, 77; and exercise, 133; and grilling meat, 44; insoluble fibre, 31; and phytochemicals, 20, 108; and soybeans, 62

candy, 93, 118

canola oil, 12

carbohydrates:
   beans, 61; calories per gram, 9; grains, 30

carrots, 20, 25

cataracts, and antioxidants, 19

catechins, 108

cereals:
   bars, 89; fibre content, 37–8; as snacks, 92; sweetened, 38

cheese, 13
   fresh, 75; grams of fat, 76; as snacks, 92

chemicals, in food supply, 27–8, 48–9

chestnuts, grams of fat, 70

chicken:
   cooking tips, 49; grams of fat, 48; ground, 47, 48

chickpeas, 63, 65

children:
   and caffeine, 106; and eating, 157–63; fat requirement, 13–14; fibre, 34; overweight, 129, 134;

snacking, 86; and vegan diets, 82–3

chili, 65–6

chocolate, 12, 27, 96–7

cholesterol:
   eggs, 57; and seafood, 53; and shrimp, 53; sources of, 11

citrus fruits, and phytochemicals, 20

CLA (conjugated linoleic acid), 77

clams, 56

Coca-Cola, sugar per serving, 153

coconut oil, 12

coffee, 102, 105–8
   decaffeinated, 105; withdrawal, 107

colon cancer, high-fibre foods, 31

constipation, and insoluble fibre, 31

convenience foods, 143–7

cookies, about, 99–100

copper. *See* trace minerals

corn oil, 12

cottage cheese, 80

crackers, 89

cranberry juice, 25

cream cheese, grams of fat, 36

croissants, 40

cruciferous vegetables, 21

desserts, 95–100
   children, 160; fast food, 155; fruit, 26–7; grams of fat, 96

diabetes, and exercise, 133

dieting:
   and children, 160; chronic, 130; difficulties, 129–30

diets, and nutrition, 128

dining out, 147–51

dogs, and exercise, 136

doughnuts, grams of fat, 40

drug, alcohol as a, 113

eggplant, and fat, 18

eggs, 57–9
   and cholesterol, 57–8; grams of fat, 58

energy level, and snacking, 86

exercise:
   benefits, 133–6; and weight loss, 132

fast food, 152–6
   grams of fat, 152

fats, 9–12
   calories per gram, 8; and children, 158; daily gram quota, 13–14; and grains, 30; sources of, 14

fatty acids, 8, 51

fibre, 18, 31–4
   beans, 62; daily intake, 33; and satiety, 130

fish, 51–5, 144
   cooking tip, 53; frozen, 54; grams of fat, 53; how to buy, 55

flatulence, and beans, 63–4

flavonoids, 108

flaxseed, 31

flour, about, 36

fluoride, in water, 104

folic acid, 18, 30, 69, 140

food safety, 55–6

free radicals, 19, 108, 111

French toast, 40

frozen foods:
   dinners, 145–6; fish, 54; fruits, 26, 98; vegetables, 26; yogurt, 91, 97–8

fruits, 17–23
   adding to diet, 22; dark green and orange rule, 19, 20; dessert, 98–9; fats in, 9; grams of fat, 18; as snacks, 92; top ten, 21

gastrointestinal problems, and yogurt, 75

genistein, 62

goat's milk, 78

grains, 41
   fats in, 9; grams of fat, 30; Mediterranean diet, 29; servings, 34

granola, 38
   bars, 89

HDL (good cholesterol), 11–12, 111
health, and fish, 52
heart disease:
  and antioxidants, 19; and exercise, 133; and phytochemicals, 20, 108; and saturated fat, 7–8
heart health:
  and fats, 9, 10; and fish, 51–2; frequent meal plan, 86–7; and meat, 43; nuts, 70; soluble fibre, 31; and wine, 110–11
heartburn, and coffee, 107
high blood pressure:
  and potassium, 121; and salt, 120–1
honey, 36
hummus, 65
hunger, and eating, 129
hydration tips, 102–3
hydrogenated fat, 10
hypertension. *See* high blood pressure

ice cream, 98
immune system, and yogurt, 75
infant formula, 77
insoluble fibre, 31
  beans, 62; sources of, 33
iron, 44, 82, 137–8, 140
  and grains, 30; nuts, 69
isoflavones, 62

jams and jellies, 36
juices, 25
  vitamin C, 38

labelling:
  beef, 45; calories from fat, 13, 14; cholesterol, 12; dietary fibre, 33; fruit drinks, 25; fruit sugars, 117; ground meats, 47; hamburger patties, 47; "light" or "lite", 9; "low in fat", 9; milk, 76; pasta, 39; salt, 123; sodium, 122; sugar, 116, 118; tofu, 66; vegetable oil, 10, 11
lactose intolerance, 78
LDL (bad cholesterol), 11–12
lead, in tap water, 103
"light", meaning of, 71
linseed oil, 31

McDonald's, grams of fat, 153, 154, 155
mad cow disease (BSE), 49
magnesium, 18, 30, 69, 73
margarine, 13
  and butter, 11; grams of fat, 36
mayonnaise, fat in, 14
meat, 43–9
  lean, 44–7; processed, 44, 46–7; to tenderize, 46

microwave:
  potatoes, 145; vegetables, 23
milk, 73–6
  calories from fat, 76; chocolate, 74; and colds, 78; cow's versus goat's, 78; daily requirement, 79; as snacks, 92
milk products:
  grams of fat, 76, 77; misconceptions, 77–9
mineral supplements, 137–8
monounsaturated fats, 9
  nuts, 70; peanut butter, 36; sources of, 10
muffins, 40–1, 91
  grams of fat, 40
mussels, 56

niacin, 44, 138
nutraceuticals, 138
Nutrasweet, 119
nutrition tips, 144, 145, 146
nuts:
  fats in, 9; grams of fat, 69–70; nutrients in, 69; as snacks, 92

oat bran, 32
oils:
  fats in, 9; heart-healthy, 12
olive oil, 9, 12
omega-3s, 12, 51–2
osteoporosis:
  and calcium, 73–4; and exercise, 133
oysters, 56

palm oil, 12
pancakes, 40
Parmesan cheese, grams of fat, 77
pasta, and sauce, 38–9
peanut butter, 13, 70
  grams of fat, 36; natural versus commercial brands, 71; as snacks, 92
pesticides, in food, 27–8
pets, and healthy owners, 136
phosphorus, 73
physical activity, and weight loss, 132
phytates, 62
phytochemicals, 20–1
  in grains, 30; in red wine, 111; in tea, 108
phytoestrogens, 62, 63
pizza, 145, 154
Pizza Hut, grams of fat, 154
polyphenols, 108, 111
polyunsaturated fats, 9
  sources of, 10
popcorn, 89–90
pork, grams of fat, 46

potassium, 18, 69, 73
  and high blood pressure, 121
potato chips, 88
pregnancy:
  and alcohol, 113; and caffeine, 106–7; fish and essential fats, 52; and sugar substitutes, 119
pretzels, 90
processed foods, saturated fats in, 9
processed meats, 44, 46–7
prostate cancer, and soybeans, 62
protease inhibitors, 62
protein:
  beans, 61; milk, 73; sources, 44
psyllium, 31–2

ramen noodles, 39
"Rate Your Weight" chart, 127
recipes, The Best of the Best Recipes index, 220
refried beans, 66
restaurants, eating in, 148
resveratrol, 111
riboflavin, 73
rice, 39
rice cakes, 90

salad dressing, fat in, 14, 25
salads:
  bean, 66; convenience foods, 143; and fat, 154; in restaurants, 24
salt:
  canned beans, 65; canned vegetables, 26; convenience foods, 143; fast food, 152; fish high in, 55; and high blood pressure, 120–1; land mines, 122; in prepackaged foods, 40, 120; pretzels, 90; processed cheese, 80; processed meat, 46; substitutes, 122; in vegetable juices, 25
sandwiches, 23, 92–3
saponins, 62
saturated fats, 7, 9
  and cholesterol levels, 57; meat, 44; and seafood, 52; sources of, 8, 10
seafood, 51–6
  grams of fat, 53; and saturated fat, 52
seeds, fats in, 9
serving sizes:
  beans, 64; eggs, 59; fruits, 22; grains, 34; meat, 44–5; milk products, 79; nuts, 70; vegetables, 22
shellfish:
  nutrition tip, 56; and safety, 55–6
sherbets, 98
shrimp:
  and cholesterol, 53; serving tip, 54
sleep, and coffee, 106

snacking, 85–93
  approach to, 87; children, 160
snacks, grams of fat, 89
sodium, 120, 122
soft drinks, sugar, 118
soluble fibre, 31–2
  beans, 62; sources of, 33
sorbets, 98
soups, 146
  and dieting, 130; as snacks, 92; and vegetables, 24
soy milk, 62, 78
soy products, 67
soybeans, fat content, 62
spreads, for bread, 36
stir-fries, 26, 145
storage:
  fruits and vegetables, 22; tomatoes, 24
sugar:
  calories in, 115; as fat substitute, 118; myths, 116–18; substitutes, 118–19
sulforaphane, 21
sunflower oil, 12
sushi, about, 55
Swiss Chalet, grams of fat, 153, 154

tap water:
  safety of, 103; taste, 104
tartar sauce, lower-fat, 54
tea, 102
  health benefits, 108–10; herbal, 110
television:
  and children, 161; and overweight, 132
thiamin, 30
tofu, 62, 66
tomatoes, 23, 24
tortilla chips, 88–9
tortillas, 40
trace minerals, 18, 44
  and grains, 30; and nuts, 69
trans fatty acids, 10
tuna, 54–5
  and omega-3s, 52
turkey, ground, 47, 48

ulcers, and coffee, 107

vegan diets, 82–3
vegetables, 17–23
  adding to diet, 22–7; and children, 161–2; cooking tip, 21; dark green and orange rule, 19, 20; fats in, 9; grams of fat, 18; grilling, 26; as snacks, 93; top ten, 21
vegetarian diets, 81–3
vitamin A, 8, 18, 73, 138

vitamin B, 30, 35, 69
vitamin B6, 138
vitamin B12, 44, 73, 82, 139
vitamin C, 18, 19, 140
    and the common cold, 138; juices, 38
vitamin D, 8, 73–5, 82, 138–9
vitamin E, 8, 19, 30, 35, 138, 140

vitamins, 8, 138–9
    supplements, 137–8

waffles, 40
water, 101–4
    and air travel, 151; bottled versus tap debate, 104; eight glasses a day, 102; pollution and fish, 55

See also tap water
water systems, home treatment, 104
weight:
    and fibre, 32; healthy, 126; how to lose, 125–36
Wendy's, grams of fat, 155
whole grain products, 31, 35, 91
wine, benefits from, 110–11

workouts, and body fat, 132

yogurt, 75
    grams of fat, 76; as snacks, 93

zinc, 30, 44, 69, 73, 82, 137, 138

The Best of the Best Recipes

Alfredo à la Genovese, 197
Apples:
    -banana muffins, 170; breakfast bars, 168; cranberry clafoutis, 209; flan, 212
Asparagus, and salmon on greens, 196

Baked fish Aegean-style, 194
Bananas:
cream topping, 172; and rolled oats cake, 211
Bars, apple, 168
Basmati and red onion pilaf, 179
Beans:
    minestrone, 177; 'n' rice, 178; Tex-Mex tortilla pie, 202
Beef:
    chili, 184; with kiwifruit, 189; lasagna, 191; shepherd's pie, 193; spicy, 190
Best ever turkey chili, 184
Blueberries:
    pancakes, 172; strawberry pear crisp, 210
Broccoli:
    pesto fettuccine, 199; soup, 176; with sunflower seeds and orange, 208
Bruschetta pizza, 200
Burgers, chicken and mushroom, 187
Burritos, 198
Buttermilk, salad dressing, 174
Buttermilk oat-branana cake, 211
Butternut squash casserole, 203

Cake, banana, rolled oats and buttermilk, 211
Carrots:
    chicken and potatoes with, 186; honeyed, 204; lemon roasted, 205
Casseroles, butternut squash, 203
Cheesecake, 213
Chicken:
    cacciatore, 188; chili, 184; Dijon, 185; and mushroom burgers, 187; with potatoes and carrots, 186
Chickpeas:
    hummus, 181; shepherd's pie, 193

Chili, turkey, 184
Clafoutis, apple and cranberry, 209
Classic Fettuccine Alfredo, 197
Cod, with basil and lemon, 195
Cranberry and apple clafoutis, 209
Creamy mushroom risotto, 180
Crisp, blueberry strawberry pear, 210

Desserts:
    apple cranberry clafoutis, 209; banana and rolled oats cake, 211; blueberry strawberry pear crisp, 210; cheesecake, 213; plum flan, 212; strawberry cream mould, 214
Dips:
    hummus, 181; sun-dried tomato and parsley pesto, 182
Down under beef with kiwifruit, 189

Eggs, French toast, 171

Fettuccine:
    Alfredo shrimp, 197; broccoli pesto, 199
Fish:
    Aegean-style, 194; fillets with basil and lemon, 195
Flan:
    apple, 212; plum, 212
Flounder, Aegean-style, 194
French toast, 171

Half hour spicy beef, 190
Halibut, Aegean-style, 194
Herb buttermilk dressing, 174
Herb-roasted chicken breasts with garlic, potatoes and carrots, 186
Honeyed carrots, 204
Hummus dip with tortilla snackers, 181

Italian pilaf, 179

Kidney beans:
    chili, 184; and rice, 178; tortilla pinwheels, 183

Lasagna, 191
Lemon roasted potatoes, 205

Liz's poppy seed vinaigrette, 173

Make-ahead baked French toast, 171
Maple mashed sweet potatoes, 207
Marinades:
    for beef, 189, 190; tofu, 200
Minestrone soup, 177
Modern mashed potatoes, 206
Mozzarella cheese:
    burritos, 198; lasagna, 191; Tex-Mex tortilla pie, 202
Muffins:
    apple-banana, 170; pineapple-carrot wheat, 169
Mushrooms:
    and chicken burgers, 187; risotto, 180; and tomatoes with penne, 201

Noodles, with spicy beef, 190

Orange ginger dressing, 196

Pancakes, blueberry, 172
Parsley pesto, 182
Pear blueberry strawberry crisp, 210
Penne with tomatoes, mushrooms & basil, 201
Perch, Aegean-style, 194
Pesto:
    broccoli, 199; parsley, 182
Pilaf, 179
Pineapple-carrot wheat muffins, 169
Pizza, bruschetta, 200
Plum flan, 212
Poppy seed vinaigrette, 173
Pork tenderloin with roasted sweet potatoes, 192
Potatoes:
    chicken and carrots with, 186; lemon roasted, 205; modern mashed, 206; shepherd's pie, 193

Refried beans, burritos, 198
Rice:
    and beans, 178; pilaf, 179; risotto, 180
Risotto, 180
Rolled oats, buttermilk-banana cake, 211

Salad dressing:
    herb buttermilk, 174; orange ginger, 196; poppy seed vinaigrette, 173
Salads:
    salmon on greens, 196; sweet potato, 175
Salmon:
    with basil and lemon, 195; on greens, 196
Sesame-crusted salmon on greens, 196
Shepherd's pie with garlic mashed potatoes, 193
Shrimp and garlic fettuccine Alfredo, 197
Soups:
    broccoli, 176; minestrone, 177
Spicy mashed sweet potatoes, 207
Squash casserole, 203
Strawberry:
    blueberry pear crisp, 210; cream mould, 214
Sun-dried tomato and parsley pesto dip, 182
Sunflower seed and orange broccoli, 208
Sweet potatoes:
    lemon roasted, 205; with pork tenderloin, 192; salad, 175; spicy mashed, 207

Tex-Mex tortilla pie, 202
Tofu:
    bruschetta pizza, 200; marinated, 200
Tomatoes, penne with mushrooms and, 201
Tortillas:
    bean pinwheels, 183; burritos, 198; Tex-Mex pie, 202
Tropical pilaf, 179
Turkey, chili, 184

Vegetables, minestrone, 177
Vinaigrette, poppy seed, 173